T0324077

Contemporary Islamic Perspectives in Public Health

"This book is an essential resource for healthcare professionals and academics seeking to deepen their understanding of the cultural nuances that shape the health and well-being of Muslim communities. With its thorough exploration of Islamic beliefs and practices related to healthcare, the authors provide invaluable insights into culturally competent care to equip practitioners with the knowledge and tools needed to promote positive health outcomes. It is a must-read for anyone involved in public health, medicine, social work, or policymaking, offering practical strategies and interventions that bridge cultural divides and enhance patient care in Muslim contexts."

Associate Professor Zuleyha Keskin
Associate Head of School, Centre for Islamic Studies and Civilisation,
Charles Sturt University, Australia

Contemporary Islamic Perspectives in Public Health

Edited by

Basil H. Aboul-Enein
University of Massachusetts Dartmouth and London School of Hygiene & Tropical Medicine

G. Hussein Rassool
Charles Sturt University

Nada Benajiba
Ibn Tofail University

Joshua Bernstein
A.T. Still University of Health Sciences

MoezAllslam E. Faris
Applied Science Private University

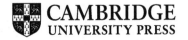
CAMBRIDGE
UNIVERSITY PRESS

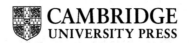

Shaftesbury Road, Cambridge CB2 8EA, United Kingdom

One Liberty Plaza, 20th Floor, New York, NY 10006, USA

477 Williamstown Road, Port Melbourne, VIC 3207, Australia

314–321, 3rd Floor, Plot 3, Splendor Forum, Jasola District Centre,
New Delhi – 110025, India

103 Penang Road, #05-06/07, Visioncrest Commercial, Singapore 238467

Cambridge University Press is part of Cambridge University Press &
Assessment, a department of the University of Cambridge.

We share the University's mission to contribute to society through the pursuit of
education, learning and research at the highest international levels of excellence.

www.cambridge.org
Information on this title: www.cambridge.org/9781009231251

DOI: 10.1017/9781009231268

First published 2025

A catalogue record for this publication is available from the British Library

*A Cataloging-in-Publication data record for this book is available from the
Library of Congress*

ISBN 978-1-009-23125-1 Paperback

Contents

Contributors

Sawsan Mustafa AbdallaSuliman
Majmaah University, Saudi Arabia

Mohammad Abdullah
Markfield Institute of Higher
Education, UK

Basil H. Aboul-Enein
Health and Society Program, College
of Arts & Sciences, University of
Massachusetts Dartmouth; Faculty of
Public Health and Policy, London School
of Hygiene & Tropical Medicine

Howeida Hassan Abusalih
Department of Health Sciences, College of
Health and Rehabilitation Sciences,
Princess Nourah bint Abdulrahman
University, Saudi Arabia

Samah Alageel
Community Health Sciences Department,
College of Applied Medical Sciences, King
Saud University, Saudi Arabia

Mohammed Ali Albar
International Medical Center,
Saudi Arabia

Maha H. Alhussain
Department of Food Science and Nutrition,
College of Food and Agriculture Sciences,
King Saud University, Saudi Arabia

Fatmah Almoayad
Department of Health Sciences, College of
Health and Rehabilitation Sciences,
Princess Nourah bint Abdulrahman
University, Saudi Arabia

Ied Shukur Alnidawi
College of Arts and Sciences, Abu Dhabi
University, United Arab Emirates

Noura Alomair
Community Health Sciences Department,
College of Applied Medical Sciences, King
Saud University, Saudi Arabia

Ahmed S. BaHammam
Department of Medicine, University Sleep
Disorders Center and Pulmonary Service,
King Saud University, Saudi Arabia; The
Strategic Technologies Program of the
National Plan for Sciences and Technology
and Innovation in the Kingdom of Saudi
Arabia, Saudi Arabia

Huny Mohamed Amin Bakry
Faculty of Medicine, Zagazig
University, Egypt

Nada Benajiba
Regional Designated Center of Nutrition
AFRA/IAEA, Ibn Tofaïl University –
CNESTEN, Morocco

Hasnae Benkirane
Regional Designated Center of Nutrition
AFRA/IAEA, Ibn Tofaïl University –
CNESTEN, Morocco

Joshua Bernstein
College of Graduate Health Studies, A.T.
Still University, MO, USA

Amina Bouziani
Regional Designated Center of Nutrition
AFRA/IAEA, Ibn Tofaïl University –
CNESTEN, Morocco

Hassan Chamsi-Pasha
GNP Hospital, Saudi Arabia

Mustapha Diaf
Faculty of Life and Natural Science,
Department of Biology, Djillali Liabes

University, Algeria; Laboratoire de Nutrition, Pathologie, Agro-Biotechnologie et Santé (Lab-NuPABS), Algeria

Elizabeth Dodge
College of Professional Studies, University of New England, ME, USA

MoezAllslam E. Faris
Department of Clinical Nutrition and Dietetics, Faculty of Allied Medical Sciences, Applied Science Private University, Amman, Jordan

Howieda Fouly
Faculty of Nursing, Assuit University, Egypt

Yasmine Guennoun
Regional Designated Center of Nutrition AFRA/IAEA, Ibn Tofaïl University – CNESTEN, Morocco

Neama Y. Hantira
College of Nursing Jeddah, King Saud University for Health Sciences, Saudi Arabia; Faculty of Nursing, Alexandria University, Egypt

Nour Horanieh
Department of Family and Community Medicine, College of Medicine, King Saud University, Saudi Arabia

Husameldin Elsawi Khalafalla
Department of Health Education and Promotion/ Institute of Nutrition and Translational Research in Metabolism, Faculty of Health, Medicine and Life Sciences, Maastricht University, Maastricht, The Netherlands

Meghit Boumediene Khaled
Faculty of Life and Natural Science, Department of Biology, Djillali Liabes

University, Algeria; Laboratoire de Nutrition, Pathologie, Agro-Biotechnologie et Santé (Lab-NuPABS), Algeria

Amal I. Khalil
Faculty of Nursing, Menoufia University, Egypt; College of Nursing, King Saud University for Health Sciences, Saudi Arabia

Lana Faiz Mahrous
Department of Health Sciences, College of Health and Rehabilitation, Princess Nourah bint Abdulrahman University, Saudi Arabia

Dheen Mohamed M. Meerasahib
College of Islamic Studies, Hamad Bin Khalifa University, Qatar

Noura Mostafa Mohamed
Faculty of Medicine, Department of Medical Biochemistry, Zagazig University, Egypt; Department of Basic Health Science, Foundation Year, Princess Noura bint Abdelrahman University, Saudi Arabia

Khaled Obaideen
Sustainable Engineering Asset Management (SEAM) Research Group, University of Sharjah, United Arab Emirates

Janine Owens
Faculty of Biology, Medicine and Health, School of Health Sciences, University of Manchester, UK

G. Hussein Rassool
Centre for Islamic Studies & Civilisations, Charles Sturt University, Australia

Eman Hassan Waly
Faculty of Medicine, Zagazig University, Egypt

About the Editors

Dr. Basil H. Aboul-Enein is an assistant teaching professor at the University of Massachusetts at Dartmouth and a distance-learning tutor of public health at the London School of Hygiene & Tropical Medicine in the UK. Dr. Aboul-Enein has previously worked in several academic institutions and previously served as a medical intelligence officer in the United States Air Force. His more than 95 publications focus on topics covering global health issues, public health historiography, public health nutrition, cultural competency in health education, medical humanities, and international health (with a focus on the Middle East and North Africa).

Dr. G. Hussein Rassool is the Professor of Islamic psychology at the Centre for Islamic Studies & Civilisations at Charles Sturt University in Australia. He is a leading academic in the areas of Islamic psychology and psychotherapy. He has published over 22 books and over 120 papers and reviews in peer-reviewed journals.

Dr. Nada Benajiba is currently an associate researcher and independent consultant in the field of nutrition. Based at the Regional Designated Center of Nutrition AFRA/IAEA at Ibn Tofaïl University – CNESTEN in Morocco, she is involved in nutrition and public health with an emphasis on cultural components in Arab countries. She is also actively involved in promoting research and leadership capacity-building in nutrition across Africa.

Dr. Joshua Bernstein is an associate professor in the Doctor of Education in Health Professions Program at the College of Graduate Health Studies at A.T. Still University in Missouri, USA. He has a PhD in health education and an MA in education, is a certified health education specialist, and is a certified wellness specialist.

Dr. MoezAlIslam E. Faris is Professor in the Department of Clinical Nutrition and Dietetics, Faculty of Allied Medical Sciences, Applied Science Private University, Amman, Jordan. He is one of the top authors of Ramadan fasting research. He has previously authored *Foods of the Holy Qur'an: A Modern Scientific Perspective*, the first scientific book that amalgamates the sacred Holy Qur'anic texts on food and nutrition with contemporary scientific knowledge.

Acknowledgments

The editors would like to extend their utmost gratitude to all the chapter authors that joined us in this book project. Without their shared expertise, knowledge, and dedication, this edited book would not have come to fruition. This expertise, knowledge, and dedication stems from a sincere affection for and appreciation of a religion that was uttered from one profound word: "*Iqraa*" (Read).

Introduction to Islam

Dheen Mohamed M. Meerasahib

Introduction

Islam, one of the most rapidly spreading religions in the world, is practiced by more than a quarter of the world's population [1]. As a distinct religious entity, Islam began with the encounter of Muhammad bin 'Abd Allāh of Makkah (peace be upon him [PBUH]) (570–632 CE) with archangel Jibrīl (Gabriel) who appeared to him during his contemplative retreat in the cave of Hira on the outskirts of Makkah in 610 CE [2]. This encounter also witnessed the first revelation of God to Muhammad in which the first five verses of chapter 96 of the **Holy Qur'an** – the revealed word of God according to Muslims – were revealed.

Defining Islam and Muslim

The Arabic word *Islām* derives from the root S-L-M which denotes a variety of closely linked connotations, which we will mention separately to bring out their import. Its first most common and literal meaning is to submit, to resign, or to surrender; it is from the active participle of the fourth form of this root that we get the word "Muslim" which literally means "one who surrenders himself," in this case, to God. Submission encompasses obeying God through the principles He revealed in the Qur'an and following the example set by the Prophet Muhammad (PBUH), who is regarded as the final messenger of God and has been entrusted with the task of interpreting the final revelation to mankind (Q Al-Baqarah 2:151; Al-Qiyamah 75:17–19). Secondly, it also denotes peace and tranquility: "Anyone abiding by or submitting to the teachings of Islam attains peace and lives in peace in this world and in the hereafter" [3]. Thirdly, it means safety and security, meaning that by following the path of Islam one becomes saved in this life and the hereafter. Finally, the term Islam is used in the Qur'anic lexicon to depict the religion of all Prophets sent by God (Q Al 'Imran 3:67; Ash-Shura 42:13; An-Nisa 4:163).

A person becomes a Muslim by accepting and pronouncing the statement, "There is no god but Allah and Muhammad is Allah's messenger," a statement known in the Muslim tradition as *al-Shahadah* (literally, witnessing).

Islam views itself as a continuation of previous dispensations of God's revelation. Its sacred scripture, the Qur'an, is, as Muslims believe, the concluding chapter of divine revelation to humanity. This belief prompts Muslims to recognize two significant facets of their faith: the acknowledgment of the natural presence of other faith traditions and religions and the affirmation of Prophet Muhammad (PBUH) as the final messenger of God, thereby establishing the belief in the "finality of his Prophethood." The Qur'anic term "Seal of the Prophets" (Q Al-Ahzaab 33:40) unequivocally states this truth, and

Muslim theology takes it to be a foundational criterion for determining the "Muslimness" of a Muslim, meaning thereby that anyone who denies this truth ceases to be a member of the Muslim community [4].

Revelation (*wahy*) and Reason (*'aql*)

Islam establishes itself upon Divine revelation, as manifested in the Qur'an and the Sunnah of the Prophet (PBUH), and it introduces this revelation alongside human reason as the principal sources of Islamic faith and practice across all facets of human life. A harmonious interaction between reason and revelation ensures the perpetuation of divine guidance for Muslims, both individually and collectively. It is thus little wonder that the Qur'an repeatedly exhorts Muslims to think and reflect and invites them to continue the pursuit of knowledge from diverse sources in order to excel in understanding and comprehension.

For Muslims, the Holy Qur'an, with its 6,200-odd verses spread over 114 chapters, represents the final revelation of God to the Prophet (PBUH), revealed over 23 years (610–632 CE). As it came in bits and pieces, it was immediately preserved through memorization and writing in the right order under the precise instruction and guidance of the Prophet (PBUH) in his lifetime [5, 6, 7].

The Sunnah of the Prophet (PBUH) denotes his sayings, actions, tacit approvals, and behavioral patterns and plays the three-fold role of a) interpreting the Holy Qur'an, b) carrying a distinctive legislative function, and c) providing the model *par excellence* worthy of emulation by Muslims. This role of the Sunnah has been clearly defined in the Qur'an itself: "*And We have sent down the Reminder unto thee that thou mightest clarify for mankind that which has been sent down unto them, that haply they may reflect*" (Q An-Nahl 16:44); "*Whatsoever the Messenger gives you, take it; and whatsoever he forbids to you, forgo, and reverence God*" (Q Al-Hashr 59:7); "*It is not for a believing man or a believing woman, when God and His Messenger have decreed a matter, to have a choice regarding the matter. Whosoever disobeys God and His Messenger has strayed into manifest error*" (Q Al-Ahzaab 33:36).

The above verses of the Qur'an make it evidently clear that both the Qur'an and Sunnah are inseparable, and the prophetic model has been made authoritative. The Qur'an further says, "*Indeed, you have in the Messenger of God a beautiful example for those who hope for God and the Last Day, and remember God much*" (Q Al-Ahzaab 33:21). It is for this reason that the person of the prophet has been made an object of love without which the faith of the believer remains incomplete.

As for reason, it is considered a divine agent infused with "divine light" and incorporates multiple degrees of understanding [8]. Moreover, it plays a central role in understanding revelation and deriving applications that aid Muslims in meeting the challenges of time and responding to ever-new evolving life situations. Its most advanced function manifests through the exercise of *Ijtihad* (literally, striving), whose crucial hermeneutic and legislative roles in the interpretation of the Qur'an and the Sunnah and the derivation of injunctions, rulings, and guidance for the Islamic way of life, both for individuals and society, cannot be overemphasized. This exercise of *Ijtihad*, which is Islam's doorway to interaction with and exploration of new ideas and applications, led to the birth and development of methodological tools, preserved as the Science of Uṣūl al-Fiqh (Principles of Jurisprudence).

It is worth noting that Muslims, when engaged with interpretation and legislation, ensure that the process is free of rationally hostile or irrational (not to be confused with suprarational) elements, both at the level of the premises and the derived conclusions. After all, the core of Islamic epistemology itself is nothing but the constructive engagement of reason with revelation.

Understanding Islam

In approaching Islam, one must keep in mind two essential facts: one, that Islam defies all endeavors to impose on it categories foreign to it, and two, that its revelational criteria are absolute and non-negotiable. Accordingly, any attempt to understand Islam should start on its own terms, as should be the case with all religions and philosophies. To begin with, Islam introduces itself as *dīn* (loosely translated as "religion") [9], a "divinely ordered comprehensive way of life," or, as technically defined by Muslim scholars, "a divine order which is in harmony with reason and leads its followers to success and happiness in this life and in the Hereafter." It provides a worldview that inspires and guides a theological system, ethical norms and practices, legislation and rituals, culture and civilization, spirituality and eschatology, intellectual and scientific pursuit, individual and public health, and a scheme for personal and social transformation.

Ḥadīth Jibrīl

Perhaps, the most useful tool for gaining a comprehensive understanding of Islam is that which has been provided by the prophetic tradition known as Ḥadīth Jibrīl (the Prophetic tradition related to Angel Gabriel). This Hadith elaborates on the concept of religion, presenting it as a multidimensional philosophy of life intertwined with eschatology and the "signs of the time" to strengthen the believers' practical connection to this philosophy. It takes the form of a dialogue which unfolds as Angel Gabriel, appearing as a stranger whom only the Prophet (PBUH) could recognize, poses five questions to the Prophet (PBUH): "what is Islām," "what is *Imān*," "what is *Iḥsān*," "when is the Day of Judgement," and "what are its signs." The Prophet (PBUH) responded to each of his queries. After Gabriel had left, the Prophet (PBUH) disclosed to his companions, "This was Jibrīl; he came to teach you your dīn" [10]. Since the Prophet (PBUH) used the term *dīn* in his final comment on this tradition, his statement has been understood by Muslims to mean that his concept of religion encompasses the elements Angel Gabriel inquired about. Moreover, it is understood that any exploration of Islam as a religion ideally needs to start with this tradition.

Islām

The first, most evident, and exterior dimension of Islam – the religion – is submission (*Islām*). It is traditionally represented through "the five pillars of Islam." Of these, the first is the **Shahadah** (witnessing or attesting to the truth), that is, to believe that "there is no God but Allah and Muhammad (PBUH) is Allah's messenger." By pronouncing this statement, an individual becomes a full-fledged member of the Muslim community and is obliged to accept all that has been prescribed by the Holy Qur'an and the Sunnah of the Prophet (PBUH) and practice them to the best of their ability. This enactment has to be carried out by Muslims in love for Allah (Q Al 'Imran 3:31) and His

Prophet (PBUH) [10, 11] and in imitation of the excellent example of the Prophet (PBUH) (Q Al-Ahzaab 33:21). This makes love the basis of everything Islamic. The remaining four pillars are establishing daily prayers (*salah*), paying the alms (**zakat**), fasting during the month of Ramadan (*sawm*), and performing the pilgrimage (**hajj**) to Makkah if and when one is physically and financially capable of doing so [10]. While these pillars constitute foundational Islamic practices, the Shahadah embraces the whole body of **Sharia**, the Islamic guideline to all aspects of Muslims' personal and communal lives, from personal hygiene to public health, and from international relations to environmental concerns.

Īmān

The second and slightly deeper metaphysical dimension is that of *Īmān* (faith), that is, to believe in "God, His angels, His books, His messengers, the Hereafter or Day of judgment, and divine providence" [10]. The denial of any of these articles renders a Muslim unfaithful to the degree of his denial. Together, these articles largely constitute the subject matter for Islamic theological, philosophical, and spiritual studies. They also provide the basics of the theoretical worldview of Islam, which is a God-centered worldview focusing on a God who is known through certain attributes, "whose whole creation is His family" [12] and "who created Adam (the first man) in His image" [13] and made him His vicegerent to all creation (Q Al-Baqarah 2:30). He guides His most noble creation "man" to Himself through human messengers whom He handpicks, each from and to his own community and, in the case of Prophet Muhammad (PBUH), to all communities to come until the day of judgment. Most great religions share belief in these articles either partially or comprehensively, at times under externally variant yet internally similar garbs, thus rendering Islam innately poised to converse with all of them.

Iḥsān

The third dimension, *Iḥsān*, literally, doing something excellently, is defined by the Prophet (PBUH) as, "To worship God as if you see Him, if you do not see Him then He certainly sees you" [10]. Here, the Prophet (PBUH) refers to the innermost or spiritual dimension of Islam. Put simply, it refers to the condition of the heart when it becomes awakened to the reality of "perpetually living in the presence of God." As such, this aspect of Islam is almost entirely concerned with the activity of the heart, and thus it is inalienably connected to the other two dimensions and prompts Muslims to seek excellence in their faith and practice.

Historical Manifestations of Islamic Dimensions

Together, the three previously mentioned dimensions address three aspects of human behavior: bodily activity (body), discursive reasoning (mind), and activity of the heart (spirit) – or, in other words, actions, beliefs, and psychological/spiritual conditions. Early Muslim generations applied the term *fiqh* (literally, understanding), but technically understanding the true message of the Holy Qur'an and the Sunnah applies to all three dimensions. The study of the first dimension was called **Fiqh al-Jawāriḥ** (the *fiqh* of the physical rituals), the second dimension, **al-Fiqh al-Akbar** (the greater *fiqh*), and the third dimension, **Fiqh al-Qulūb** (the *fiqh* of the heart/spirit) [14]. Intellectual deliberations over the three dimensions of Islam and their application in Muslim societies organically led to the development of three broad disciplines along with several ancillary ones: a) 'Ilm al-Kalām (the science of Creed, popularly known in western academia as Islamic or Kalam Theology), b) 'Ilm al-Fiqh (the science of Law and Jurisprudence), and c) 'Ilm al-Taṣawwuf (the science of Islamic spiritual quest), respectively [15]. Later historical development led to the rise of several juristic, theological, and spiritual schools of thought in each of the above areas. Today, two large schools, the mainstream **Sunni** tradition and the smaller **Shī'ī** tradition (with their respective internal diversities) in addition to the Ibāḍīs of Oman have, however, prevailed [16].

With respect to the schools of jurisprudence among the Sunnis, four continue to enjoy eminence: **Ḥanafīs** (followers of the Persian Abū Ḥanīfah), **Mālikīs** (followers of Mālik bin Anas of Madina), **Shafi'īs** (followers of Muhammad bin Idrīs al-Shafi'ī), and **Ḥanbalīs** (followers of Aḥmad bin Ḥanbal of Iraq). As for Shī'ahs, their two prominent schools include the **Ithnā 'Asharīs/Ja'farīs** (Twelvers, after their fifth spiritual leader Ja'far al-Ṣādiq) and **Zaydīs** (after Zayd, grandson of Ḥusayn, the Prophet's grandson) [16]. As *fiqh*'s domain was bodily activities and changing life situations required continuous attention, Islamic scholarship virtually became synonymous with juristic expertise. In situations when Muslims were faced with issues where the primary sources seemed silent, jurists resorted to *Ijtihad* guided by the spirit of revelation and prophetic model to seek answers. Two foundational intellectual activities emerged in this regard – **Ijmā'** (general consensus of the scholars of a particular age) and **Qiyās** (to strive to drive appropriate rulings by logical inference and analogy) – which constitute the most renowned modes of *Ijtihad* still today [17].

Likewise, in the area of faith, or kalam, Sunnis are divided into three broad schools: **Ash'arīs** (followers of Abu'l-Ḥasan al-Ash'arī) and **Maturidīs** (followers of Abū Manṣūr al-Māturidī), who constitute the overwhelming majority of Sunnis, and a smaller **Ahl al-Ḥadīth** group (the literalists) who also survived the tides of times [18]. As for Shī'ahs, they were traditionally aligned with the rationalist **Mu'tazilīs**. Their major theological factions include the **Ithnā'Asharīs** (Twelvers), **Ismā'īlīs**, and **Zaydīs**, all of whom share and disagree on a variety of topics with Sunnis and among themselves in varying degrees.

Finally, the discipline of Taṣawwuf relates to the art of disciplining the self to help Muslims gradually progress to the level where they become and strive to remain conscious of the Divine presence at all times. The system developed to facilitate this process came to be called the *Ṭarīqah* (the way) and involved the growth of centers of spiritual guidance called *Ḥalaqāt, Ribāṭ, Khānqāh,* or *Zāwiya* in various parts of the Muslim world [19]. They functioned under the leadership of a master, who provided spiritual guidance to the **sālik/murīd** (wayfarer). Over time, *ṭarīqahs* progressed into more structured entities usually named after their founders (**Qādiriyyah, Shādhiliyyah, Naqshabandiyyah, Chishtiyyah,** and **Suhrawardiyyah,** to name a few) that continue to this day and represent the most widespread depiction of Islam.

Islam and the Rise of a Benefactor Civilization

This three-dimensional understanding of Islam along with the disciplines and institutions that developed around it remain to this day the mainstream tradition of Islam. In addition, several other disciplines of knowledge such as **'Ulūm al-Qur'an,**

'Ulūm al-Ḥadīth, Uṣūl al-Fiqh, and 'Ulūm al-Lughah were developed by Muslims to serve the purpose of scriptural reasoning and facilitate the exercise of *Ijtihad*.

The intellectual efforts of Muslim scholars were not restricted to these religious or "transmitted" sciences; rather, Muslims broke new grounds and often innovated in the fields of linguistics and literature, astronomy, geography, international relations, philosophy, psychology, ethics, governance, society, mathematics, physics, biology, botany and zoology, hydraulics, and so on. Their achievements were significant and far-reaching in their effect on subsequent human civilizations and contributed to their awakening and replenishment. Muslim scholars thus created knowledge on the one hand while also serving as a conduit of knowledge between ancient, contemporary, and later peoples [20].

After the Prophet's (PBUH) death, the Muslim community entered into a period of experimentation with respect to governance. Four rightly guided caliphs saw through the first thirty years, after which dynastic rule took over (**Ummayyads, Abbasids, Fatimids, Seljuqs,** etc.) and the Muslim world experienced periods of political fulfillment and disgrace. The **Mongol invasion** of the thirteenth century dealt a fatal political blow to the Muslim world but failed to dampen their passion for knowledge and both intellectual and scientific advancement. When the Ottomans established their caliphate, the Muslim world was able to recover some of its lost glory.

Islam as *dīn* stands faithful to a way of life that is God-centered. No separation between this world and the next is envisaged. Individuals and societies ought to be governed by the "revealed guidance" and discursive reasoning based on it. There is no bar on benefiting from the positive achievements of other cultures, provided they do not contradict the core teachings of Islam. At the same time, religious freedom is guaranteed; "*There is no compulsion in religion*" (Q Al-Baqarah 2:256) is one of the hallmarks of the Qur'anic teachings, and hence Muslims do not have the right to impose their religion on anyone. A friendly attitude towards other religions is an obligation (Q Al-Mumtahanah 60:8; Al-Hujuraat 49:13).

Islam's social philosophy is based not only on faith and the brotherhood of all humanity but also on the nurturing and purification of the individual soul. All human problems, in the final analysis, are ethical in their origin, which is why Islam accords the utmost importance to morality, so much so that the Prophet (PBUH) described the ultimate purpose of his advent as an ethical one by saying, "I have been sent to perfect the highest moral virtues" [21]. Human dignity and social responsibility are foundational, and all systems are supposed to be erected on them. Muslim social systems are inherently geared to create an environment of justice, prosperity, and social security for all – whether they are Muslims or non-Muslims. These systems are largely driven by moral precepts which are virtually incumbent upon all Muslims; these include visiting the sick, condoling family members of the deceased, caring for orphans and the poor, and so forth. This moral order plays a significant role in ensuring the preservation of the social and psychological welfare of the individual and society.

The Islamic principles of faith and practice are intertwined with the notion of safeguarding public health. Central to Islamic belief is the concept of *Tawḥīd*, or the oneness of God. This principle underscores the interconnectedness of all beings and emphasizes that all creatures belong to God alone. Consequently, Muslims are called upon to recognize the sanctity of life and to uphold practices that promote the well-being of the individual and society as a whole. Through adherence to rituals grounded in meditation, purity, and cleanliness, individuals cultivate a sense of inner peace and serenity which extends outward to their interactions with the "other."

Islam also emphasizes the importance of nurturing a harmonious relationship with nature, characterized by love, mercy, and charity. Muslims are encouraged to be stewards of the environment, recognizing that the Earth is a trust from God. This entails adopting sustainable practices and showing compassion towards all living beings. By embracing these teachings, Muslims contribute to the preservation of public health as they prioritize the protection and promotion of life in all its forms. Through acts of charity and kindness, they seek to remove suffering and promote physical, psychological, sociological, spiritual, and public health and well-being within their communities. Thus, Islam offers a holistic framework for addressing public health challenges that is rooted in principles of unity, compassion, and reverence for creation.

With the dawn of the modern era, when most Muslim lands were colonized and Muslim societies became nation-states, their fortunes began to change. The spirit of Islam dampened, and intellectual activity stalled. Muslim subjugation to the gradually dominating culture of the West, particularly in technological sciences, resulted in them forgetting their worldview. Scholars differ in the assessment of the several revivalistic efforts made by Muslims from the nineteenth century onwards as they differed in determining the cause of Muslim "stagnation and backwardness." In my opinion, however, the cause does not relate to the status of scientific progress as much as it relates to two factors foretold by the Prophet (PBUH) centuries ago: "unwarranted love of this world and abhorrence to meeting the Lord" [13], and here lies the elixir.

Further Reading

Nasr, S. H., Dagli, C. K., Dakake, M. M., & Lumbard, J. E. *The Study Quran: A New Translation and Commentary*. New York: HarperCollins Publishers. 2015.

References

1. Pew Research Center. The changing global religious landscape. [online]. 2017 [Accessed May 4, 2023]. Available from: www.pewresearch.org/religion/2017/04/05/the-changing-global-religious-landscape/

2. Hishām, I. *Sīrat Ibn Hishām*. Notes by 'Umar Abd al-Salām Tadmuriyy. Beirut: Dār al-Kitāb al-'Arabī, 1990.

3. Al-Aṣfahānī, A. R. *Mufradāt Alfāẓ al-Holy Qur'an*. Damascus: Dār al-Qalam. 2009.

4. 'Aysh, U. A. M. *'Aqīdat Khatm al-Nubuwwah bi'l-Nubuwwah al-Muḥammadiyyah*. Cairo: Maktabat al-Azhar. 1976.

5. Dā'ūd, A. Wā'iẓ, M. D., ed. *Kitāb al-Maṣāḥif*. Beirut: Dār al-Bashā'ir al-Islāmiyyah. 2002.

6. Al-A'ẓamī, M. M. *The History of the Qur'anic Text from Revelation to Compilation: A Comparative Study with the Old and New Testaments*. Leicester, UK: UK Islamic Academy. 2003.

7. Al-A'ẓamī, M. M. *The Scribes of the Prophet*. London: Turath Publishing. n.d.

8. Al-Ghazālī, A. H. *Mishkāt al-Anwār wa Miṣfāt al-Asrār*. Beirut: 'Ālam al-kutub. 1986.

9. Darāz, M. A. A. *Al-Dīn*. Kuwait: Dār al-Qalam. 1952.

10. Al-Qushayrī, M. B. H. *Saḥīḥ Muslim*. Beirut: Dār Iḥyā' al-Turāth al-'Arabī. n.d.

11. Al-Bukhārī, M. B. I. *al-Jāmī al-Ṣaḥīḥ*. Beirut: Dār Ṭawq al-Najāt. 2001.

12. Al-Bayhaqī, A. B. *Shu'ab al-Īmān*. Beirut: Dār al-kutub al-'Ilmiyyah. 2010.

13. Ḥanbal, A. B. *Musnad Aḥmad*. Beirut: Mu'assasat al-Risālah. 2001.

14. Al-Tuwaijirī, M. B. I. *Mawsū'at al-Fiqh al-Islāmī*. Amman: Bayt al-Afkār al-Dawliyyah. 2009.

15. Zarrūq, A. *Ightinām al-Fawā'id fī Sharḥ Qawā'id al-'Aqā'id*. Kuwait: Dār al-Diyā'. n.d.

16. Zahrah, Abū. Introduction. In: Bashā, A. T., ed. *Naẓrah Tārīkhiyyah fī Ḥudūth al-Madhāhib al-Fiqhiyyah al-arba'ah*. Beirut: Dār al-Qādirī. 1990.

17. Ḥasaballah, A. *Uṣūl al-Tashrī' al-Islāmī*. Cairo: Dār al-Ma'ārif. 2006.

18. Al-Shaṭṭī, H. *Mukhtaṣar Lawāmi' al-Anwār al-Bahiyyah*. Damascus: Maṭba'at al-Taraqqī. 1931.

19. Nasr, S. H. Preclude: the spiritual significance of the rise and growth of the Sufi orders. In: Nasr, S. H., ed. *Islamic Spirituality: Manifestations*. New York: The Crossroad Publishing Company. 1997.

20. Nasr, S. H. *Science and Civilization in Islam*. Chicago: ABC International Group, Inc. 2001.

21. Al-Bayhaqī, A. B. *al-Sunan al-Kubrā*. Beirut: Dār al-kutub al-'Ilmiyyah. 2003.

The Qur'an and Prophetic Guidance: An Overview in the Context of New Public Health

G. Hussein Rassool, Janine Owens

Introduction

This chapter gives an overview of the emergence of New Public Health (NPH), including the challenges of its scientific development, and focuses on health promotion in the context of Islam. The chapter suggests that the evidence base needs to shift from the discipline's biomedical roots towards a cohesive integration of the practices and beliefs of Muslim communities.

Emergence and Global Relevance of NPH

Some authors suggest that Western perceptions of public health lie in the physiocratic thinking of ancient Greece during the sixth through fourth centuries BCE in defining health as a state of dynamic equilibrium between the internal and the external environment [1]. Later, following a parliament-sanctioned investigative commission, Sweden provided data to investigate the underlying causes of the increase in poverty, inequality, mass urbanization, worker safety, and poor housing from 1840 to 1920 [2]. This early focus on research and statistics by the commission provided the foundation for what we now know as epidemiology and contributed to the formation of the Swedish welfare state [2]. Other authors argue that the concept of public health emerged during the Industrial Revolution, in the nineteenth century, when John Snow traced the origins of the 1854 cholera epidemic in London to a water pump in Broad Street [3]. After this came the development of environmental sanitation, the focus on disease reduction, and the major achievement of public health resulting from the provision of clean water through chlorination and filtration processes [3, 4, 5].

The successful development of public health in high-income countries and its advances in reducing the incidence of communicable diseases led to alternative ways of thinking about health, focusing more on the social environment, and the realization of the complexity in which it operates, which eventually led to a conceptual development called "New Public Health" (NPH) [6].

New Public Health is an integrative approach to preventing and promoting the health of populations, and it is constantly evolving [7]. It currently encompasses a wide range of preventive, curative, and rehabilitative factors that are crucial to health and well-being [8, 9]. In particular, the 1986 introduction of the Ottawa Charter for Health Promotion [10], built on the Alma-Ata Declaration of 1978, identified primary health care as the key to the attainment of the goal of "Health for All" [8]. The general agreement within the public health community was to base the move from health protection to health promotion on the Ottawa Charter principles, and this constituted NPH [11, 12]. The Ottawa Charter for

Health Promotion proposed five key aims: building healthy public policy, creating supportive environments, strengthening community action, developing personal skills, and reorienting health services [10]. While the focus on the social determinants of health [13] and inequalities [14] as well as a move away from the medicalization of health and the introduction of other disciplines such as sociology [15] are positive strengths, one downside to this proposition is that the five key areas of health promotion are only workable in high-income countries (HICs) where piloting originally occurred [16, 17]. This is primarily because HICs have well-developed, strongly governed, and accountable public health systems and low population growth. The populations of many low- and middle-income countries (LMICs) are rapidly expanding, and the architecture of their health systems varies. Therefore, governance and delivery of health systems depends on country-specific government roles, mandates, and actions. This means that some systems are decentralized and are the responsibility of regional author-ities, offering the flexibility to respond to local needs but simultaneously creating challenges for addressing failures around referrals and the care continuum. This is mainly because providers at higher-level facilities do not share the same reporting structure as those at lower-level facilities. Workers at community, primary health, and district levels often report through and to different leadership structures compared to secondary care or tertiary hospitals. Therefore, referrals and care pathways may be incomplete, suboptimal, and fragmented. Furthermore, measurement of performance enables the tracking of progress and development of health systems in order to drive improvement and create accountability. Low- and middle-income countries exhibit significant data gaps, and the absence of clear measures constrains improvement efforts and limits accountability and the ability to focus health improvement efforts [18]. For example, in some LMICs, the absence of data is even more severe with no basic registration data for births, deaths, or pregnancies. The lack of clear measurement led in part to the global health community prioritizing vertical programs because tracking key interventions over time (such as vaccination, malaria control, tuberculosis, and HIV) provided evidence of progress [18]. The Millennium Development Goals grew out of this approach with variable levels of success and a legacy of fragmented health systems which focused on treating specific diseases rather than implementing comprehensive health promotion [18]. This complexity in LMICs leaves a vertical and disease-focused approach to health and a focus of funding on hospitals and tertiary care due to communicable diseases that affect the immediate health needs of the population [19]. In LMICs, fewer resources and under-developed or non-existent public health systems create a narrow focus and concentrate government attention and resources on communicable diseases and tertiary health care, creating challenges for many aspects of public health practice [19]. Although noncommunicable diseases such as obesity, cancer, cardiovascular disease, and so on are present and increasing in LMICs alongside population growth, the existing challenges of reducing communicable diseases in these expanding populations appears to leave NPH in its infancy. Therefore, while HICs with more organized, accountable, and advanced public health systems can measure and focus on noncommunicable diseases, for LMICs healthy public policy, health promotion, scaling up services, and advocacy, as proposed by the Ottawa Charter for Health Promotion, [10] may lag behind because they have less developed and accountable public health systems, data gaps, an absence of clear measurement, fewer resources, rapidly expanding populations, and burgeoning health needs resulting from the impact of communicable and noncommunicable diseases.

Global austerity further affects population health, which was exacerbated by COVID-19 and the resulting pressure on already constrained health and social care services. New Public Health reflects societies, their inherent power structures, socioeconomic development, and cultural understandings [8], but it fails to include religion and spirituality in its thinking. This is because of the way NPH, medicine, and psychiatry developed, each splitting away from religion and spirituality [20]. However, the focus on physical health also creates a further divide from mental health with a lack of parity between the two and a subsequent rise in health inequalities [21]. New Public Health tends to draw on different disciplines – for example, medicine, epidemiology, psychology (behavioral accounts of health), sociology, and anthropology (cultural accounts of health). The prominence of physical health over mental health within medicine has sidelined religion and spirituality, which in turn reduces the evidence base for NPH. More recently, the move towards patient-centered care in medicine shifts the focus towards religion and spirituality as being part of a whole-patient approach to care instead of merely focusing on disease.

New Public Health, Religion, and Spirituality

Numerous publications now link religion, spirituality, and health, but despite this increasing connection these areas receive little consideration in NPH compared to the disciplines of sociology and nursing [22]. The influence of religious and spiritual beliefs and practices on health may sometimes exert negative effects – for example, cultural perceptions about practices such as female genital mutilation and cutting (FGMC) [23]. This is where complexity arises because the effect of culture becomes intrinsically bound to religion and spirituality even though FGMC is not a religious practice. Therefore, while unpicking the nature of the relationship may assist in the introduction of improvements, there is also a remaining cultural tension. However, religious and spiritual beliefs can exert positive effects, such as those found in the nine-year longitudinal study by Berkman and Syme that focused on men and women aged 30–69 attending temple or church in the USA. In this study, they explored the impact that social support, religion, and spirituality have on socioeconomic status and health behaviors such as smoking, alcohol use, physical inactivity, obesity, and low utilization of preventive health services [24]. The study found that religion, spirituality, and social support are protective factors against a wide range of disease outcomes, although it could not explain the mechanisms by which these networks influence health [24]. Apart from the protective dimension of religion and social support, other studies find positive associations between religious prayer and coping with stress and other mental health difficulties [25]. A recent systematic review identified that spiritual community participation is associated with healthier lives, greater longevity, lower rates of depression and suicide, and reduced levels of substance misuse [26].

In many publications, different perceptions exist about Muslim religiosity compared to other religions, with Islam appearing either subsumed under studies including Christianity and Judaism or altogether absent [27]. For NPH, its development within a science-based approach, opposition to religious concepts, and the notion that integrating spirituality may somehow bias public health programs, [28] leaves a further gap in the evidence base about the sociocultural aspects of health and the potential impacts of faith-based health promotion.

Public Health Challenges for Different Muslim Countries

Globally, there is diversity between and within the 48 out of 190 countries that are classified as Muslim-majority countries (MMCs) including large health-related disparities linked to gross national income, literacy rates, access to clean water, health systems, and levels of corruption, creating significant health inequity for MMCs when compared to non-MMCs [29]. One point to underline here is that there is no evidence to suggest that religion is responsible for health inequity. Instead, it is the health gradient between and within countries and the inequitable distribution of power, income, services, and other structural determinants that form the social determinants of health and are responsible for the inequities in people's lives.

However, cultural diversity intertwines with religion and disparities related to the social determinants of health and different cultural perceptions, beliefs, and practices around health and illness, presenting a complex picture and creating public health challenges. Another issue is that some MMCs are developing, while others are already developed. This diversity creates more challenges for the public health workforce and for some MMCs with developing public health systems where the focus remains on communicable disease control. High-income MMCs are mostly Arab states that have a poor track record of investing in public health; data suggests that, on average, the expenditure on health in Arab states equalled just 5% of GDP, which is lower than the average for LMICs as a whole (5.4%) [30]. Inequity is also present, especially between urban and rural populations, and is dependent on age, educational level, and socioeconomic status. Then there is the issue of complex conflicts in states such as Iraq, Syria, Yemen, Libya, and the occupied Palestinian territories, which have decreased health outcomes alongside conflict-specific factors like poorly served refugee populations, attacks on health care facilities and personnel, sanctions and blockades, and high rates of mental and physical trauma, which distinguish these MMCs from their more stable neighbors [30]. Rapid population growth also places increasing pressures on health systems. While there have been investments in the health sector that have increased the number of facilities and providers, the Gulf states spend less on health care than countries with comparable development and income – 3.8% of GDP compared to a global average of 10% [30].

Further complications appear with emergent pandemics and the need for strong public health guidance, with the most recent example being COVID-19. In some countries, there is strong political support for a developed public health system with its approaches viewed as important for achieving national health goals because it focuses on promoting health and preventing noncommunicable disease, creating a distinct advantage for these populations in contrast to those in more fragile countries.

Qur'anic and Prophetic Public Health-Related Guidance

At the time of the first Islamic caliphate in the seventh century, Islam was at the forefront of the development and implementation of what we would now call public health, as evidenced by multiple indications in the primary Islamic texts. Far from being a separate discipline, medicine was part of medieval Islamic culture, with centers of learning developing from famous mosques and hospitals. Many Islamic cities had sewage systems, public baths, and clean running water at a time when Europe neglected these public health necessities. Islamic personal and public health practices developed during the seventh century still apply in modernity. Today, the majority of Muslims accept Western evidence-based medicine and receive their medical care in hospitals, but the influences of the remnants of earlier Islamic medical philosophies still remain. For example, *tibb al-nabi*, or prophetic medicine, comprises health information contained in the Qur'an, Hadith, and Sunnah of the Prophet Muhammad (PBUH). Prophetic medicine does not distinguish between physiological and psychological illness. Although Muslims use Western health care in high-income Muslim countries, they still use traditional herbal medicines described in the Qur'an such as black seed, garlic, and myrrh [31].

Islam is a holistic belief system and does not subscribe to the Cartesian duality (or the mind–body divide) present in Western medicine; health is one construct and is not segregated into physical and mental health. Therefore, embedded within the construct of health are the dimensions of physical, psychological, emotional, and spiritual well-being or positive health. Islam prioritizes health, placing it second in importance to faith. The divine law contains the five essential needs for living: faith, life, progeny, property, and mind, and "60% of these essentials (three out of the five), namely life, progeny, and mind, cannot be adequately safeguarded without the protection and preservation of health" [32 p. 1]. A suggestion is that emphasizing prevention within Islamic public health messages enables it to be "included in the whole discourse of good decisions in daily living, from eating to cleanliness and taking appropriate precautions" [33 p. 1]. The Hadith (a collection of traditions containing sayings of the Prophet Muhammad [PBUH] which, with accounts of his daily practice [the Sunnah], constitutes the major source of guidance for Muslims apart from the Qur'an) reflects the promotion of public health.

For example, the Qur'an guides child development, recognizing the importance of breastfeeding in the seventh century, but the modern-day mantra of "breast is best" would have placed less pressure on women then compared to today because of the acceptability of wet nurses:

> And the mothers should suckle their children for two whole years for him who desires to make complete the time of suckling; . . . if both desire to wean by mutual consent and counsel, there is no blame on them, and if you wish to engage a wet-nurse for your children, there is no blame on you so long as you pay what you promised for according to usage; and be careful of (your duty to) Allah and know that Allah sees what you do.
>
> (Q Al-Baqarah 2:233)

From 2017 to 2018, researchers employed a nutritional intervention in a Qur'an pilot program utilizing religious leaders as key agents of change in five communities (Nikerabad, Charshanbe, Meserabad, Jalalabad, and Eraghli) in the Sheberghan District, Jawzjan Province, Afghanistan [34]. The pilot demonstrated the potential for integrating public health nutrition messaging with Qur'anic guidance in Afghanistan. Furthermore, the authors argued that easy adaptation, replication, and scaling up of the study is possible in other Islamic countries because the nutrition messages identified adhere to the Qur'an and the Hadith.

Another example from the Qur'an is the promotion of healthy eating in adults: "*Eat of the good things we have provided for your sustenance, but commit no excess therein, lest my wrath should justly descend on you, and those on whom descends my wrath do perish indeed*" (Q Ta-Ha 20:81). Refraining from overindulgence could reflect the NPH plate portion approach to weight control; furthermore, the Sunnah of Prophet David (PBUH) recommends fasting every other day. This reflects recent thinking on the 5:2 diet which facilitates weight loss and reduces cardiovascular risk; disproportionate weight gain (or obesity) and its impact on cardiovascular health are both risk factors for type 2 diabetes [35]. However, the oil-rich MMCs of the Arabian Gulf – Bahrain, Kuwait, Oman, Qatar, Saudi Arabia, and the United Arab Emirates (UAE) – are a distinct group. Due to the financial stability acquired from their natural resources, they have undergone the epidemiological transition at faster rates than their regional neighbors. Physically demanding labor is relegated to migrants, and the exceedingly high temperatures encourage citizens of these countries to stay inside, causing a move towards sedentary lifestyles. Easy access to unhealthy foods, such as fast food chains and other elements of Western diets, further contributes towards noncommunicable diseases such as obesity and type 2 diabetes, which occurs in more than 60% of citizens across the Gulf states and is the leading cause of morbidity and mortality for some MMCs [36]. Paradoxically, although nutritional and dietary changes have occurred in some MMCs, political and economic problems in other MMCs affect food availability – for example, the current conflicts in Gaza in the occupied Palestinian territories and Syria, as well as recurrent famine in Somalia.

The sexual and reproductive rights of adolescents and girls is a global priority, and although there is guidance on sexual health in the Qur'an, for MMCs these are often overlooked because of the conservative cultural context that prohibits sexual activity outside marriage [37]. The influx of refugees to Jordan due to the conflict in Syria has impacted reports from Jordan, which indicate a 10.7% rise in displaced adolescent girls marrying under the age of 18, some as young as 12, with the accompanying problems of early pregnancy, intimate partner violence, poor mental health, and loss of future opportunities [38].

Historical documents such as the Qur'an and the oral traditions of the Hadiths (prophetic sayings) are viewed as eternal; therefore, the past exerts an influence on the present, making it indistinguishable. For example, social quarantine is not a twenty-first-century NPH innovation to protect people from death, sickness, and epidemics or pandemics like COVID-19. Over 1,400 years ago, the Caliphate of Prophet Muhammad (PBUH), probably after observing plague outbreaks, advised on the concept of quarantine, instructing his companions to adhere to preventive behaviors. Allah's Messenger (PBUH) referred to the principles of modern quarantine when he wrote, "If you hear about it (an outbreak of plague) in a land, do not go to it; but if the plague breaks out in a country where you are staying, do not run away from it" [39]. This is about the prevention and control of disease and follows a contagion approach to health prevention, which did not occur until the nineteenth century in Europe. The basis for the practices of social quarantine and social distancing parallel principles derived from the advice of the Prophet (PBUH). Another Hadith reports God's Messenger (PBUH) as saying, "Flee from one who has tubercular leprosy as you would from a lion" [40] to prevent the spread of airborne droplets, bacteria, and viruses. This follows the miasmic theories of infection, present up to the nineteenth century, and Abu Hurairah discusses the health-related practices of the Prophet (PBUH) narrating that when he sneezed he would "cover his face with his hand or with his garment and muffle the sound with it" [41].

The Qur'an places great emphasis on cleanliness and personal hygiene. Allah the Almighty says: "Indeed, Allah loves those who are constantly repentant and loves those who purify themselves" (Q Al-Baqarah 2:222). Cleanliness is both a physical and spiritual act, and Islam insists on several practices to facilitate this process. Within the Hadith the Messenger of Allah (PBUH) echoes the importance of cleanliness. Abu Malik at-Ash'ari reported that the Messenger of Allah (PBUH) said, "Cleanliness is half of faith" [42]. This emphasizes the intertwined nature of spirituality and health-related practices. Another Hadith from the Prophet Muhammad (PBUH), Abu Hurairah, narrated that "the Messenger of Allah (PBUH) said: And Allah loves those who make themselves clean and pure" [43]. Prior to engaging in the five daily prayers, Muslims must carry out *wudu* (washing with clean water). Further, cleansing the whole body from impurities (*Ghusl*) is encouraged at least weekly. Undertaking *Ghusl* also occurs after acts of intimacy, childbirth, post-natal bleeding, menstruation, and when preparing the deceased for burial. The Prophet Muhammad (PBUH) also guided Muslims to wash their hands before preparing and eating food: "The blessing of food consists in ablution before it and ablution after it" [44]. These examples from the Qur'an illustrate that it contains Islamic practices and guidance focusing on a holistic conception of health to guide a Muslim, both spiritually and practically, throughout the course of life.

Linkages to New Public Health

Islam reveres health as a fundamental human right of every human being, reflecting the rights-based approach of New Public Health. The Hadith and Sunnah of the Prophet Muhammad (PBUH) parallel guidance in New Public Health but follow a more saluto-genic approach, focusing on factors that support human health and well-being rather than on those causing disease [45]. Salutogenesis means the "origin of health," and within this model people have general resilience resources (GRRs) enabling them to conceptualize the world as organized, understandable, and meaningful. Islam enables Muslims to organize their worlds and gives them meaning. GRRs are the internal and external resources people use to cope with stressors and play an important role in the ways they perceive challenges throughout life. The ability to use these resources is called sense of coherence (SOC). Islam is a GRR because it provides Muslims with a way of overcoming challenges, guided by their faith in Allah. SOC occurs through mindfulness along with Islamic principles and practices as a way of navigating people's daily lives. Whatever happens is because Allah means it to happen. This belief is both positive and negative when reflecting on noncommunicable diseases because fatalistic approaches to health can affect help-seeking behaviors and may influence the view that preventive actions have no influence on health outcomes. Stripping back the negativity means returning people to basic Islamic principles, which stipulate that a human body is a gift from Allah and as such requires looking after.

Recent uses of Islamic principles and practices may be found in place-based health promotion, where health education takes place in mosques and framing health messages alongside scriptural sources effectively promotes health practices and knowledge in Muslim populations [46]. However, one concern that emerged is the credibility of the person giving the message, who in this case is the imam at the mosque. The imam is male, but women felt that female health messages, because of their personal and private nature, should be given by a female.

Conclusion

Islamic health care practices and guidance emerged over 1,400 years ago within the Qur'an and Hadith and predate public health. Islam considers the body holistically for

Muslims globally, viewing health and spirituality as one and linking health-related beliefs and practices using a salutogenic focus. However, NPH struggles in MMCs and LMICs because of numerous complexities, such as poorly resourced and accountable systems, the health gradient between and within countries, inequitable distribution of power, income, and services, as well as other structural determinants. There are also complex conflicts in some MMCs which contribute to health inequalities. Further, there is the rise of noncommunicable diseases in some high-income MMCs, which increases the complexity of health care. New Public Health is in its infancy for some countries and therefore tends to retain its focus on communicable disease and primary health care because it is easier to measure successful outcomes. Incorporating Qur'anic guidance into health-promoting messages in NPH may assist in developing and extending its reach, simultaneously creating sustainable health promotion interventions for Islamic communities.

References

1. Tountas, Y. The historical origins of the basic concepts of health promotion and education: the role of ancient Greek philosophy and medicine. *Health Promotion International*. 2009;24 (2):185–92. https://doi.org/10.1093/ heapro/dap006

2. Irwin, R. Sweden's engagement in global health: a historical review. *Globalization and Health*. 2009;15(1): 79. https://doi .org/10.1186/s12992-019-0499-1

3. Tulchinsky, T. H. John Snow, cholera, the Broad Street pump: waterborne diseases then and now. In: *Case Studies in Public Health*. Cambridge, MA: Academic Press. 2018. 77–99. https://doi.org/10.1016/ B978-0-12-804571-8.00017-2

4. Rosen, G. *From Medical Policy to Social Medicine: Essays on the History of Health Care*. New York: Science History Publications. 1974.

5. Porter, D., ed. *The History of Public Health and the Modern State.* Amsterdam: Editions Rodopi BV. 1994.

6. Frenk, J. The New Public Health. *Annual Review of Public Health*. 1993;14:469–90. https://doi.org/10.1146/annurev.pu.14 .050193.002345

7. Beaglehole, R. & Bonita, R. *Public Health at the Crossroads: Achievements and Prospects*. 2nd ed. Cambridge: Cambridge University Press. 2004.

8. World Health Organization, Regional Office for Europe. *Declaration of Alma Ata*. 1978. Available from: https://iris.who .int/handle/10665/347879

9. Lawn, J. E., Rohde, J., Rifkin, S., Were, M., Paul, V. K., & Chopra, M. Alma-Ata 30 years on: revolutionary, relevant, and time to revitalise. *The Lancet*. 2008;372:917–27. https://doi.org/10.1016/ s0140-6736(08)61402-6

10. World Health Organization, Regional Office for Europe. *Ottawa Charter for Health Promotion, 1986*. 1986. Available from: https://iris.who.int/handle/10665/ 349652

11. Baum, F. *The New Public Health: An Australian Perspective*. Oxford: Oxford University Press. 1998. 12–21.

12. Wills, J. *Practicing Health Promotion: Dilemmas and Challenges*. London: Bailliere Tindall. 1998. 18–24.

13. Solar, O. & Irwin, A. A conceptual framework for action on the social determinants of health. In: *Discussion Paper Series on Social Determinants of Health*, No. 2. Geneva: World Health Organization. 2010. Available from: www .who.int/publications/i/item/ 9789241500852

14. Naik, Y., Baker, P., Ismail, S., Tillmann, T., Bash, K., Quantz, D., et al. Going upstream: an umbrella review of the macroeconomic determinants of health and health inequalities. *BMC Public*

Health. 2019;19:1678. https://doi.org/10.1186/s12889-019-7895-6

15. Awofeso, N. What's new about the "new public health"? *American Journal of Public Health*. 2004;94(5):705–9. https://doi.org/10.2105/ajph.94.5.705

16. Awofeso, N. The Healthy Cities approach: reflections on a framework for improving global health. *Bulletin of the World Health Organization*. 2003;81:222–23.

17. Awofeso, N., Ritchie, J., & Degeling, P. Problems and prospects of implementing the Health Promoting Schools concept in Northern Nigeria. *Health Promotion Journal of Australia*. 2000;10:164–69.

18. OECD, World Health Organization, & World Bank Group. *Delivering Quality Health Services: A Global Imperative*. Geneva: World Health Organization. 2018. https://doi.org/10.1787/9789264300309-en

19. Tulchinsky, T. H. & Varavikova, E. A. What is the "New Public Health"? *Public Health Reviews*. 2010;32:25–53. https://doi.org/10.1007/BF03391592

20. Koenig, H. G. Religion, spirituality, and health: the research and clinical implications. *ISRN Psychiatry*. 2012;2012:278730. https://doi.org/10.5402/2012/278730

21. Owens, J., Lovell, K., Brown, A., & Bee, P. Parity of esteem and systems thinking: a theory informed qualitative inductive thematic analysis. *BMC Psychiatry*. 2022;22(1):650. https://doi.org/10.1186/s12888-022-04299-y

22. Oman, D. Elephant in the room: why spirituality and religion matter for public health. In: Oman, D., ed. *Why Religion and Spirituality Matter for Public Health*. Cham: Springer. 2018. 1–16.

23. Abidogun, T., Ramnarine, L. A., Fouladi, N., Owens, J., Abusalih, H. H., Bernstein, J., et al. Female genital mutilation in Arab League states and Arabic-speaking communities: a systematic review of preventive interventions. *TMIH*. 2022;27(5):468–78. https://doi.org/10.1111/tmi.13749

24. Berkman, L. F. & Syme, S. L. Social networks, host resistance, and mortality: a nine-year follow-up study of Alameda County residents. *American Journal of Epidemiology*. 1989;109(2):186–204. https://doi.org/10.1093/oxfordjournals.aje.a112674

25. Pargament, K. I. Religion and coping: the current state of knowledge. In: Folkman, S., ed. *The Oxford Handbook of Stress, Health, and Coping*. New York: Oxford University Press. 2011. 269–88.

26. Balboni, T., VanderWeele, T., Doan-Soares, S., Long, K., Ferrell, B., Fitchett, G., et al. Spirituality in serious illness and health. *JAMA*. 2022;328(2):184–97. https://doi.org/10.1001/jama.2022.11086

27. Lance, D. L., de Marrais, J., & Barnes, L. L. Portraying Islam and Muslims in MEDLINE: a content analysis. *Social Science and Medicine*. 2007;65(12):2425–39. https://doi.org/10.1016/j.socscimed.2007.07.029

28. Addiss, D. G. Spiritual themes and challenges in global health. *J. Med. Humanit*. 2018;39(3):337–48. https://doi.org/10.1007/s10912-015-9378-9

29. Beaglehole, R. & Dal Poz, M. R. Public health workforce: challenges and policy issues. *Human Resources for Health*. 2003;1(1):4. https://doi.org/10.1186/1478-4491-1-4

30. Asi, Y. M. Health care in the Arab world: outcomes of a broken social contract. [online]. 2020 [Accessed March 26, 2024]. Available from: https://arabcenterdc.org/resource/health-care-in-the-arab-world-outcomes-of-a-broken-social-contract/

31. Weber, A. S. Clinical applications of the history of medicine in Muslim-majority nations. *Journal of the History of Medicine and Allied Sciences*. 2023;78(1):46–61. https://doi.org/10.1093/jhmas/jrac039

32. Islam, H. T., Sadia, S., Rabia, S., Khan, W., Muhammad, A., & Awan, T. A. Ethics of healthy discipline from Islamic point of view. *Journal of Positive School Psychology*. 2022;6(8):10714–19.

33. El-Hamdoon, O. H. Islam and public health. *Journal of British Islamic Medical Association.* 2021;8(3):50–53.

34. Sultani, N. & Ferdous, T. Nutrition in Qur'an: an innovative approach to promote optimal nutrition care practices. [online]. 2020 [Accessed April 3, 2024]. Available from: www.ennonline.net/fex/nutritioninquran

35. Brown, J. E., Mosley, M., & Aldred, S. Intermittent fasting: a dietary intervention for prevention of diabetes and cardiovascular disease? *British Journal of Diabetes and Cardiovascular Disease.* 2013;13(2):68–72. https://doi.org/10.1177/1474651413486496

36. Rahim, H. F, Sibai, A., Khader, Y., Hwalla, N., Fadhil, I., Alsiyabi, H., et al. Non-communicable diseases in the Arab world. *The Lancet.* 2014;383 (9914):356–67. https://doi.org/10.1016/S0140-6736(13)62383-1

37. Sahbani, S., Al-Khateeb, M., & Hikmat, R. Early marriage and pregnancy among Syrian adolescent girls in Jordan: do they have a choice? *Pathogens and Global Health.* 2016;110(6):217–18. https://doi.org/10.1080/20477724.2016.1231834

38. UNICEF. A qualitative study on the underlying social norms and economic causes that lead to child marriage in Jordan: developing an actionable multisectoral plan for prevention. [online]. 2019 [Accessed March 27, 2024]. Available from: www.unicef.org/jordan/media/1796/file/Jordan-Reports.pdf

39. Sahih al-Bukhari. *Sahih al-Bukhari 5729.* In-book reference: Book 76, Hadith 44. Available from: https://sunnah.com/bukhari/76

40. Mishkat al-Masabih. *Mishkat al-Masabih 4577.* In-book reference: Book 23, Hadith 61. Available from: https://sunnah.com/mishkat:4577

41. Jami' at-Tirmidhi. *Jami' at-Tirmidhi 2745.* In-book reference: Book 43, Hadith 15. Available from: https://sunnah.com/tirmidhi/43

42. Sahih Muslim. *Sahih Muslim 223.* In-book reference: Book 2, Hadith 1. Available from: https://sunnah.com/muslim/2

43. Sunan Ibn Majah. *Sunan Ibn Majah 357.* In-book reference: Book 1, Hadith 91. Available from: https://sunnah.com/ibnmajah/1

44. Mishkat al-Masabih. *Mishkat al-Masabih 4208.* In-book reference: Book 21, Hadith 46. Available from: https://sunnah.com/mishkat:4208

45. Antonovsky, A. *Unraveling The Mystery of Health: How People Manage Stress and Stay Well.* San Francisco: Jossey-Bass Publishers. 1987.

46. Vu, M., Muhammad, H., Peek, M. E., & Padela, A. I. Muslim women's perspectives on designing mosque-based women's health interventions: an exploratory qualitative study. *Women & Health.* 2018;58(3):334–46. https://doi.org/10.1080/03630242.2017.1292344

Islamic Applications towards Public Health Policies: A Brief Perspective

Amal I. Khalil, Neama Y. Hantira, Howieda Fouly

Introduction

Public health is defined as the science and art of preventing diseases, improving quality of life, and promoting health and efficiency through organized community efforts. Public health, along with primary care, secondary care, and tertiary care, is part of a country's overall health care system. These are sciences that serve the health of people and are considered as part of the interdisciplinary health sciences. Public health science encompasses a wide range of disciplines, including epidemiology, biostatistics, and management of health services. Public health is also one of the efforts organized by society to protect, promote, and restore people's health [1].

The Meaning of Public Health and Its Policies from an Islamic Perspective

Public health refers to the collective efforts aimed at preventing disease, promoting health, and prolonging life within a community [1]. In Islam, public health is a shared responsibility and is viewed as a way to fulfill the religious duty of preserving human life [2]. Islamic teachings emphasize the importance of hygiene, sanitation, and disease prevention. For instance, the Prophet Muhammad (PBUH) stated, "Cleanliness is half of faith" [3]. In addition, Islamic history provides examples of public health policies, such as the quarantine measures implemented during the bubonic plague outbreak in the seventh century [4]. Today, Muslim-majority countries continue to implement public health policies that are in line with Islamic teachings. For example, the Malaysian government has implemented a national health policy that includes measures to promote healthy lifestyles and prevent diseases [5].

Health Promotion: Islamic Historical Evolution

Health promotion is deeply rooted in Islamic teachings and has been emphasized throughout history. Islam highlights the importance of maintaining good health and well-being, encouraging individuals to adopt healthy lifestyles [6, 7]. Muslim physicians and scholars, such as Ibn-Sina and Al-Zahrawi, have made significant contributions to medicine and health care. Their works, including *The Canon of Medicine* and *Kitab al-Tasrif*, have had a lasting impact on medical knowledge and practice. The integration of health promotion within Islamic principles has played a crucial role in promoting health and preventing diseases [8].

Muslim-majority countries have implemented various health promotion strategies and programs to promote healthy lifestyles and prevent chronic diseases as observed in

Arabic-speaking countries [9]. Islam emphasizes the importance of individuals taking care of their physical, mental, and spiritual health, avoiding harmful behaviors, and maintaining a balanced lifestyle [10]. These principles align with contemporary health promotion efforts aiming to improve overall well-being and prevent diseases [11].

Islamic Health Policies

Throughout history, Muslim scholars and leaders have actively advocated for public health, with Prophet Muhammad (PBUH) highlighting the importance of cleanliness and implementing measures such as establishing a quarantine system [12]. These examples demonstrate the proactive approach of Islamic teachings towards maintaining and promoting public health. Hospitals and medical schools were established during the Islamic Golden Age, providing free health care regardless of social or economic status [13]. Presently, Muslim-majority countries implement Islamic health policies, including national health care systems and health promotion programs. Islamic health policies recognize health care as a basic human right, accessible to all [14]. The Qur'an emphasizes seeking medical treatment and the belief in Allah as the ultimate healer. Overall, Islamic health policies prioritize good health, disease prevention, and quality health care, contributing to the well-being of individuals and communities [15].

The Public Health Prevention Program in Islam

Islam promotes public health prevention programs and emphasizes the importance of disease prevention and health promotion. The Prophet Muhammad (PBUH) emphasized prevention in maintaining good health [16]. Throughout history, Islamic societies have implemented public health prevention programs, such as establishing hospitals and clinics [17]. Islamic teachings provide guidance on holistic health promotion, cleanliness, and preventive measures [18]. The Qur'an and Hadith emphasize moderation in consumption, cleanliness, and hygiene practices [18]. For instance, the Qur'an states, "*And eat and drink, but be not excessive. Indeed, He likes not those who commit excess*" (Q A'raf 7:31), highlighting the importance of moderation in food and drink consumption for overall health. Prophet Muhammad (PBUH) also emphasized the significance of health and hygiene. He advised his followers to maintain cleanliness and encouraged practices such as performing ablution (*wudu*) before prayers, which includes washing the hands, face, and feet [19]. Additionally, the Prophet Muhammad (PBUH) recommended preventive measures such as quarantine to contain infectious diseases [16]. He stated, "If you hear of an outbreak of plague in a land, do not enter it; but if the plague breaks out in a place while you are in it, do not leave that place" [16].

Communicable Diseases in Islam

In Islam, the control of communicable and pandemic diseases involves individual or group fatwas (religious rulings) as well as global organizational decisions. Three strategies are employed: quarantine and social distancing to prevent the spread of the disease, proper treatment of diseased cases, and respectful management of the deceased [20]. Historical examples, such as the plague of Shirawayh during the lifetime of Prophet Muhammad (PBUH), demonstrate the implementation of quarantine measures [21]. Treatment can be complemented by religious acts while acknowledging the importance of medical treatment alongside prayers and supplications to Allah [22, 23]. Fatwas have been issued to support quarantine measures and provide guidance on the treatment of the ill and the handling of deceased bodies, considering the principles of Sharia [24]. Fatwas related to health promotion offer guidance to Muslims on health matters, aligning with Islamic principles and the higher objectives of Sharia, helping individuals and communities make informed decisions and adopt preventive measures [25].

Before issuing the COVID-19 vaccine, the injection of the plasma of recovered COVID-19 patients was used to boost individual immunity. However, this measure created unregulated markets; therefore, Al-Azhar's International Center for Electronic Fatwa issued a fatwa stating that it is impermissible and sinful for recovered COVID-19 patients to withhold their plasma without a valid excuse [26]. Additionally, specific protocols were implemented for handling the deceased during the COVID-19 pandemic, which included procedures for washing, shrouding, offering prayers, burial, and providing consolation. According to the European Council for Fatwa and Research (ECFR), dead infected individuals should be buried without washing to reduce the spread of infection. Additionally, the funeral prayer can be performed in person or absentia, either individually or as a congregation [27].

Islamic Evidence-Based Research on the Effect of Climate Change

Climate change is projected to have severe health impacts, leading to an estimated 250,000 additional deaths annually by 2030–50, particularly in areas with weaker health care systems [28]. Consequently, Islamic leaders have proposed and adopted an Islamic Declaration on Climate Change and the promotion of "Islamic environmentalism" [29].

Islamic teachings emphasize environmental conservation and human responsibility to protect the natural world. Islamic scholars have issued statements and fatwas stressing the importance of environmental preservation and climate change mitigation. Islam teaches that humans are stewards on Earth with a responsibility to care for the environment and promote ecological balance and sustainable resource management. Islam emphasizes trust and responsibility towards future generations and prohibits corruption and destruction on Earth [30]. The Islamic Declaration on Climate Change calls for urgent action based on Islamic ethical principles, highlighting the importance of environmental preservation and climate change mitigation for the well-being of all creatures and future generations [31].

Public Health Policies and Culture

When considering Islam and its applications to public health policies, several important aspects should be highlighted:

Islamic Principles: Islam promotes health preservation, cleanliness, and disease prevention as vital for individual and community well-being.

Public Health Practices: Islamic teachings encourage healthy habits, including regular handwashing, proper sanitation, and maintaining a clean environment, aligning with modern public health principles.

Community Support: Islam places an emphasis on community and social responsibility, fostering support and care for one another, especially during public health crises, which aids in implementing effective public health interventions [32].

Ethical Considerations: Islamic ethics prioritize the preservation of life and the well-being of individuals and communities, providing a foundation for shaping public health policies [33].

Health Education: Islamic institutions and leaders play a significant role in disseminating health-related information, raising awareness, promoting healthy behaviors, and addressing misconceptions within Muslim communities [34].

All these aspects demonstrate how Islamic principles and values contribute to the development and implementation of effective public health policies and practices, encompassing health promotion, disease prevention, community support, ethical considerations, and health education.

Conclusion

Islam promotes public health policies that prioritize disease prevention and the promotion of good health and well-being. Islamic culture values diversity and has made significant contributions to various fields. Intercultural mediation is essential for promoting harmony and resolving conflicts in a multicultural world. Islamic education emphasizes critical thinking, moral development, and community service while fostering acceptance of diversity and promoting interfaith dialogue. The contributions of Muslims throughout history highlight the importance of intercultural exchange and cooperation. By promoting intercultural understanding and respect, society can become more inclusive and harmonious.

References

1. White, F. Primary health care and public health: foundations of universal health systems. *Medical Principles and Practice.* 2015;24(2):103–16. https://doi.org/10.1159/000370197

2. Rassool, G. H. The crescent and Islam: healing, nursing and the spiritual dimension. Some considerations towards an understanding of the Islamic perspectives on caring. *Journal of Advanced Nursing.* 2000;32:1476–84. http://doi.org/10.1046/j.1365-2648.2000.01614.x

3. Sahih Muslim. *Sahih Muslim 223.* In-book reference: Book 2, Hadith 1. Available from: https://sunnah.com/muslim:223

4. Tognotti, E. Lessons from the history of quarantine, from plague to influenza A. *Emerging Infectious Diseases.* 2013;19(2):254–59. https://doi.org/10.3201/eid1902.120312

5. Ministry of Health Malaysia. National strategic plan for non-communicable disease 2016–2025. [online]. 2017 [Accessed May 12, 2023]. Available from: www.moh.gov.my/moh/resources/Penerbitan/Rujukan/NCD/National%20Strategic%20Plan/FINAL_NSPNCD.pdf

6. Alimohammadi, N., Jafari-Mianaei, S., Bankipoor-Fard, A. H., & Hasanpour, M. Laying the foundations of lifelong health at the beginning of life: Islamic perspective. *Journal of Religion and Health.* 2020;59(1):570–83. https://doi.org/10.1007/s10943-017-0470-5

7. Sahih Muslim. *Sahih Muslim 91a.* In-book reference: Book 1, Hadith 171. Available from: https://sunnah.com/muslim:91a

8. Lakhtakia, R. A trio of exemplars of medieval Islamic medicine: Al-Razi, Avicenna and Ibn Al-Nafis. *Sultan Qaboos University Medical Journal.* 2014;14(4): e455–59.

9. Samara, A., Andersen, P. T., & Aro, A. R. Health promotion and obesity in the Arab Gulf states: challenges and good practices.

Journal of Obesity. 2019;2019:4756260. https://doi.org/10.1155/2019/4756260

10. Guntur, M. Al-Quran teach the importance of taking care of health physical: Tafseer Surat Al-Baqarah. *AKADEMIK: Jurnal Mahasiswa Humanis*. 2021;1(2):50–58. https://doi.org/10.37481/jmh.v1i2.228

11. Aboul-Enein, B. H. Health-promoting verses as mentioned in the Holy Quran. *Journal of Religion and Health*. 2016;55 (3):821–29. https://doi.org/10.1007/s10943-014-9857-8

12. Amin, J. Quarantine and hygienic practices about combating contagious disease like COVID-19 and Islamic perspective. *Journal of Critical Reviews*. 2020;7(13):3698–705.

13. Hajar, R. The air of history part III: The Golden Age in Arab Islamic medicine an introduction. *Heart Views*. 2013;14 (1):43–46. https://doi.org/10.4103/1995-705X.107125

14. Almalki, M., Fitzgerald, G., & Clark, M. Health care system in Saudi Arabia: an overview. *Eastern Mediterranean Health Journal*. 2011;17(10):784–93. https://doi.org/10.26719/2011.17.10.784

15. BinTaleb, A. & Aseery, A. What can the Prophet Muhammad teach us about pandemics? *Journal of Religious and Theological Information*. 2022;21(1–2):82–94. https://doi.org/10.1080/10477845.2021.2017552

16. Tulchinsky, T. H. & Varavikova, E. A. A history of public health. In: Tulchinsky, T. H. & Varavikova, E. A., eds. *The New Public Health*. Amsterdam: Elsevier Science. 2014. 1–42.

17. Piwko, A. M. Islam and the COVID-19 pandemic: between religious practice and health protection. *Journal of Religion and Health*. 2021;60(5):3291–308. https://doi.org/10.1007/s10943-021-01346-y

18. Koehrsen, J. Muslims and climate change: how Islam, Muslim organizations, and religious leaders influence climate change perceptions and mitigation activities. *WIREs Climate Change*. 2021;12:e702. https://doi.org/10.1002/wcc.702

19. Sahih Muslim. *Sahih Muslim 251a*. In-book reference: Book 2, Hadith 54. Available from: https://sunnah.com/muslim:251a

20. Dols, M. W. Plague in early Islamic history. *Journal of the American Oriental Society*. 1974;94(3):371–83. https://doi.org/10.2307/600071

21. Shabana, A. From the plague to the coronavirus: Islamic ethics and responses to the COVID-19 pandemic. *Journal of Islamic Ethics*. 2021;5:1–37. https://doi.org/10.1163/24685542-12340060

22. Awaad, R., Nursoy-Demir, M., Khalil, A., & Helal, H. Islamic civilizations and plagues: the role of religion, faith and psychology during pandemics. *Journal of Religion and Health*. 2023;62(2):1379–93. https://doi.org/10.1007/s10943-023-01765-z

23. Fahmy, K. *In Quest of Justice: Islamic Law and Forensic Medicine in Modern Egypt*. Oakland: University of California Press. 2018.

24. Sachedina, A. *Islamic Biomedical Ethics Principles and Application*. Oxford: Oxford University Press. 2009.

25. Buḥayrī, Aḥmad. Fatwā min al-Azhar bi-Sha 'n Tabarruʿ al-Mutaʿāfīn min Kurūnā bi-l-Bilāzmā. [online]. Al-Maṣrī al-Yawm. 3 June 2020 [Accessed March 2, 2022]. Available from: www.almasryalyoum.com/news/details/1984276

26. ECFR. Al-Mustajaddāt al-Fiqhiyya li-Nāzilat Fayrūs Kurūnā COVID-19. [online]. 2020 [Accessed July 15, 2020]. Available from: https://bit.ly/4dh3CqY

27. Lugten, E. & Hariharan, N. Strengthening health systems for climate adaptation and health security: key considerations for policy and programming. *Health Security*. 2022;20(5):435–39. https://doi.org/10.1089/hs.2022.0050

28. Jenkins, W., Berry, E., & Kreider, L. B. Religion and climate change. *Annual Review of Environment and Resources*. 2018;43(1):85–108. https://doi.org/10.1146/annurev-environ-102017-025855

29. Aboul-Enein, B. H. "The earth is your mosque": narrative perspectives of environmental health and education in the Holy Quran. *Journal of Environmental Studies and Sciences.* 2018;8:22–31. https://doi.org/10.1007/s13412-017-0444-7

30. *Islamic Declaration on Global Climate Change.* 2015. Available from: https://islamicclimatedeclaration.org/islamic-declaration-on-global-climate-change/

31. Padela, A. I., Killawi, A., Heisler, M., Demonner, S., & Fetters, M. D. The role of imams in American Muslim health: perspectives of Muslim community leaders in Southeast Michigan. *Journal of Religion and Health.* 2011;50 (2):359–73. https://doi.org/10.1007/s10943-010-9428-6

32. Akrami, F., Karimi, A., Abbasi, M., & Shahrivari, A. Adapting the principles of biomedical ethics to Islamic principles and values in the context of public health policy. *Journal for the Study of Religions and Ideologies.* 2018;17(49):46–59.

33. Mustafa, Y., Baker, D., Puligari, P., Melody, T., Yeung, J., & Gao-Smith, F. The role of imams and mosques in health promotion in Western societies: a systematic review protocol. *Systematic Reviews.* 2017;6(1):25. https://doi.org/10.1186/s13643-016-0404-4

Chapter 4

Islamic Prayer (Salat) and Health

Janine Owens

Introduction

There are five pillars of Islam, which form the framework for the lives of all Muslims. These five pillars are primary obligations. They are *Shahadah* (the creed or declaration of faith), salat or *salah* (prayer), *sawm* (fasting), hajj (pilgrimage), and zakat (charity).

Narrated Ibn "Umar"

Allah's Messenger (PBUH) said,

> Islam is based on (the following) five (principles):
> 1. To testify that none has the right to be worshipped but Allah and Muhammad (PBUH) is Allah's Messenger.
> 2. To offer the (compulsory congregational) prayers dutifully and perfectly.
> 3. To pay Zakat (obligatory charity or alms to the poor).
> 4. To perform Hajj (Pilgrimage to Mecca at least once in the lifetime of an individual).
> 5. To observe fast during the month of Ramadan. [1]

Muslims across the world unite in prayer at five specified times of the day in exactly the same way, in Arabic and, when possible, in a congregation in a mosque in the vicinity. The Prophet Muhammad (PBUH) indicated that "the prayer in congregation is twenty-seven times superior to the prayer offered by person alone" [2]. Praying in congregation unites Muslims into one cohesive community.

In the Holy Qur'an, the Arabic word *salat* means to demonstrate servitude to God by means of certain actions. Praying occurs while facing the Ka'bah (literally translated to "cube"), which is a stone building in the center of Islam's most important mosque and holiest site – the Masjid al-Haram in the holy city of Mecca in Saudi Arabia. It is considered by Muslims to be the *Bayt Allah* (House of God) and a means of connecting to Allah and the Muslim's purpose in life – to remember and worship Him.

The obligatory prayers occur five times a day, at *Fajar* (dawn), *Zuhar* (noon prayer), *Asar* (afternoon), *Maghrib* (sunset prayer), and *Ishaa* (night prayer).

The five appointed times for salat to be performed during the day are commanded in the Holy Qur'an: "*Verily, Salah is an obligation on the believers to be observed at its appointed time*" (Q An-Nisa 4:103). Meeting for congregational prayers five times a day also enables Muslims to be responsive to the needs of each other, establishing a model of social support and integration [3].

For Muslims with mobility impairments unable to leave their beds while hospitalized, turning their beds towards Mecca for prayer and making the Qur'an readily available accommodates and assists with adherence to their spiritual and religious beliefs [4].

Prayers and preparation for prayer play a central role in Muslim religious practices. Although there are other prayers – for example, self-purification prayers – performing salat is mandatory for Muslims.

Prayer and Physical Health

Salat is both a physical prayer and a type of meditation [5], comprising of a certain number of repetitive physical and spiritual units or cycles called rak'ah. salat consists of 17 mandatory rak'ah during the day, accompanied by supplications recited in Arabic. There are also 12 nonobligatory Sunnah. Prior to engaging in salat, Muslims must carry out *wudu* (washing with clean water) to purify themselves physically and spiritually. The rak'ah begins when the worshiper initiates the prayer with the words "Allahu Akbar" or God is great. In Arabic, this is the *Takbeer* (The Glorification of God), and it reminds Muslims that nothing and no one is greater than Allah, commanding their humility. At the end of salat, the person turns the head to both shoulders, first to the right and then to the left. This reminds Muslims of the presence of the recording angels on their right and left shoulders who record their deeds [6, 7].

Cycles of rak'ah consist of a series of movements while reciting sections of the Qur'an from memory, improving cognitive recall. For example, the individual tucks in their chin and looks at their feet while standing, resulting in flexion at the upper cervical spine [7]. Holding the back and head flat and perpendicular to the legs occurs for 5 to 10 seconds, and forward bending occurs at the thoracic and lumbar spine, which leads to stretching of the paraspinal muscles and structures [8]. During prostration or *sujud* (prostrating to Allah), flexion occurs at the thoracic and lumbar spine alongside hip flexion, and slight extension of the lower cervical spine occurs during prostration [6]. While *Tahiyyat* or sitting with the legs folded beneath the body for 20 to 30 seconds occurs, the lumbar and thoracic spine are in a neutral position with the hip joint in flexion and the knee joint in full flexion, resulting in the stretching of the quadriceps femoris muscle [7]. During salat, movement occurs for nearly every joint in the body, with the different postures and positions responsible for the contraction and relaxation of numerous muscles, creating an anaerobic workout that extends and flexes the muscles and joints similarly to yoga [9, 10].

Although the expectation is to perform the rak'ah during salat, Islam allows flexibility in the positions for prayer during illness. The Prophet Muhammad (PBUH) said, "Pray while standing and if you can't, pray while sitting and if you cannot do even that, then pray lying on your side" [11]. Performing rak'ah benefits people physically and mentally, stretching muscles and joints and improving cognitive recall through repetition while focusing the mind in the form of meditation. The number of rak'ah performed differs throughout the day at the appointed times.

At *Fajar* (dawn), two cycles of rak'ah are performed, at *Zuhar* (noon prayer), four rak'ah, at *Asar* (afternoon), four rak'ah, at *Maghrib* (sunset prayer), three rak'ah, and at *Ishaa* (night prayer), four rak'ah.

Physically, the movements of the rak'ah exercise the majority of joints and muscles in the body. One study argues that repetitive movements throughout the day reduce the risk of blood pooling when sedentary, assisting in the reduction of the risk of deep vein thrombosis [8]. Other studies suggest that physical actions during salat lower the heart rate and decrease diastolic and systolic blood pressure, benefiting mildly hypertensive individuals [12, 13]. The rak'ah movements strengthen the spine and neck muscles, contributing towards improving sensory information and balance in older age [3, 14, 15]. Stroke patients also benefit from performing salat in terms of balance and exercising limbs, which prevents muscle atrophy [16]. Other studies demonstrate that salat is capable of mimicking desirable pro-immune and pro-metabolic health effects [15, 17]. Evidence further suggests that regular practice of salat for Muslims results in decreased chances of development of knee osteoarthritis because of the flexing and stretching of the soft tissues around the knee joint [18, 19]. However, the majority of these studies contain sample sizes too small for generalization to occur, and the beneficial physical and cognitive effects of salat are only for individuals who pray with commitment, consistency, and regularity.

The cycles of rak'ah are not merely about movement but are also about concurrent prayers and their communal aspects, which exert an effect on cognition, memory, and well-being.

Prayer and Mental Health

Concurrent prayers accompany rak'ah, recited internally or aloud. The regularity and format of prayers in Islam create structure, and Islam aims at creating balance in the life of a Muslim by enabling the individual to put matters into perspective.

Some studies consider salat to be a form of meditation because of the repetitiveness of movements and focused recitation of prayers [7, 15, 20]. Furthermore, research on mindfulness in salat suggests a significant ($p < 0.05$) difference in positive mental health among individuals who offer prayer regularly compared to those who do not pray regularly [21]. Mindfulness implies focusing on the area of importance, in this case on the importance and greatness of Allah. A more recent scoping review of the evidence base suggests that salat and supplicant praying, recitation, memorizing, and listening to the Qur'an reduces the incidence of reactive depression, stress, and anxiety [22]. However, even though Islam is about the *Ummah* or community of Muslims globally [23], only two studies in the review mentioned the impact of communal praying [24, 25], but they failed to explore this in any depth; therefore, the review argues that this produces a gap in the evidence base [22]. The review also identifies that interventions using salat to improve mental health mainly occur in non-Western countries, indicating a lack of cultural competence in Western countries when treating Muslims and the need to design health services to accommodate and address their beliefs and needs [26, 27].

In the wider evidence base on both physical and mental health for Islam and other religions, seminal work by Koenig and colleagues confirms the positive effects of religious practices, particularly for mental health [28, 29, 30]. Salat itself creates parity between physical and mental health because the physical movements occur simultaneously with the spiritual and cognitive act of praying.

Implementing Salat in Public Health

Caring for Muslim populations often provides challenges for non-Muslim providers because of a lack of cultural understanding [31, 32]. Previous research indicates a lack of consideration of faith-based approaches in promoting physical and mental health in Muslim populations [26, 33, 34]. This chapter provides evidence that salat has a positive effect on the physical and mental health of Muslims, improving well-being and even assisting with balance for people after experiencing a stroke [16]. Another study claims that salat may have protective effects and may improve cognition, lower blood lipids, and reduce the risk of developing Alzheimer's disease [35]; however, the study was too small to be generalized, ending with a call for more studies about the beneficial effects of salat. Creatively delivering holistic care and health-promoting programs for Muslims could therefore incorporate both Western biopsychosocial approaches and faith-based needs, incorporating salat and leaning towards Antonovsky's holistic perspective of salutogenesis. Salutogenesis is an interdisciplinary approach that focuses on people's resources and capacity to create health rather than on risks, ill health, and disease (pathogenesis); it is about the interaction between the individual and societal structures [36, 37]. Application of the theory can occur at an individual, a group, and a societal level. The key elements in the salutogenic development are, firstly, the orientation towards problem solving and, secondly, the capacity to use the resources available [38]. The term for the capacity to use the resources available is sense of coherence (SOC), which is a stress resource-oriented concept, focusing on resources to maintain and improve the move towards health. People develop their SOC throughout their lives, but the foundations occur in the first decades of life when people learn how to deal with life in general, as Muslims do through salat. It is about people's ability to maintain health despite stress, and it is about attitudes and behaviors [39]. There is, therefore, a close connection between SOC and mental well-being [40], which the scoping review mentioned earlier identifies [22].

Conclusion

Salat is a spiritual, a physical, and a cognitive activity with positive health benefits. It unites physical actions with spiritual intentions and cognitive beliefs, creating an environment for mindfulness and focusing on the greatness of Allah through humility, thereby reducing the significance of the human being as they submit themselves to His will. Accompanying the submission is the gentle flexing and extending of most joints and muscles in the human body, creating a physical and spiritual melding of body and mind. Public health could utilize salutogenesis and focus on health and wellness with Muslim populations by incorporating Muslim religious practices where practical, such as within physical and mental health programs, in order to create more culturally congruent and inclusive approaches.

References

1. Sahih al-Bukhari. *Sahih al-Bukhari 8*. In-book reference: Book 2, Hadith 1. Available from: https://sunnah.com/bukhari:8

2. Sahih al-Bukhari. *Sahih al-Bukhari 645*. In-book reference: Book 10, Hadith 42. Available from: https://sunnah.com/bukhari:645

3. Sayeed, S. A. & Prakash, A. The Islamic prayer (salah/namaaz) and yoga togetherness in mental health. *Indian Journal of Psychiatry*. 2013;55(Suppl.2): S224–30. https://doi.org/10.4103/0019-5545.105537

4. Boucher, N. A., Siddiqui, E. A., & Koenig, H. G. Supporting Muslim patients during advanced illness. *The Permanente Journal*. 2017;21:16–190. https://doi.org/10.7812/TPP/16-190

5. Alwasiti, H. H., Aris, I., & Jantan, A. EEG activity in Muslim prayer: a pilot study. *Maejo International Journal of Science and Technology*. 2010;4(3):496–511.

6. Doufesh, H., Ibrahim, F., Ismail, N. A., & Ahmad, W. A. W. Effect of Muslim

prayer (salat) on α electroencephalography and its relationship with autonomic nervous system activity. *Journal of Alternative and Complementary Medicine.* 2014;20 (7):558–62. https://doi.org/10.1089/acm .2013.0426

7. Doufesh, H., Ibrahim, F., Ismail, N. A., & Ahmad, W. A. W. Assessment of heart rates and blood pressure in different salat positions. *Journal of Physical Therapy Science.* 2013;25:211–14. https://doi.org/ 10.1589/jpts.25.211

8. Chamsi-Pasha, H. Islam and the cardiovascular patient: pragmatism in practice. *British Journal of Cardiology.* 2013;20(3):1–2. https://doi.org/10.5837/ bjc.2013.020

9. Safee, M. K. M., Abas, W. A. B. W., Ibrahim, F., Abu Osman, N. A., & Salahuddin, M. H. R. Electromyographic activity of the lower limb muscles during salat and specific exercises. *Journal of Physical Therapy Science.* 2012;24:549–52. https://doi.org/10.1589/ jpts.24.549

10. Bezuglov, E., Talibov, O., Butovskiy, M., Lyubushkina, A., Khaitin, V., Lazarev, A., et al. The prevalence of non-contact muscle injuries of the lower limb in professional soccer players who perform salah regularly: a retrospective cohort study. *Journal of Orthopaedic Surgery and Research.* 2020;15(1):440. https://doi.org/10.1186/ s13018-020-01955-5

11. Sahih al-Bukhari. *Sahih al-Bukhari 1117.* In-book reference: Book 18, Hadith 37. Available from: https://sunnah.com/ bukhari:1117

12. Doufesh, H., Ibrahim, F., Ismail, N. A., & Wan Ahmad, W. A. Assessment of heart rates and blood pressure in different salat positions. *Journal of Physical Therapy Science.* 2013;25:211–14. https://doi.org/ 10.1589/jpts.25.211

13. Al-Kandari, Y. Y. Religiosity and its relation to blood pressure among selected Kuwaitis. *Journal of Biosocial Science.* 2003;35(3):463–72. https://doi.org/10 .1017/s0021932003004632

14. Al-Ghazal, S. K. *Medical Miracles of the Qur'an.* Leicestershire, UK: The Islamic Foundation. 2006.

15. Alabdulwahab, S. S., Kachanathu, S. J., & Oluseye, K. Physical activity associated with prayer regimes improves standing dynamic balance of healthy people. *Journal of Physical Therapy Science.* 2013;12:1565–68. https://doi.org/10.1589/ jpts.25.1565

16. Ghous, M., Malik, A. N., Amjad, M. I., & Kanwal, M. Effects of activity repetition training with salat (prayer) versus task oriented training on functional outcomes of stroke. *Journal of Pakistan Medical Association.* 2017;67(7):1091–93.

17. Alam, I., Ullah, R., Jan, A., Sehar, B., Khalil, A. A. K., Naqeeb, H., et al. Improvement in cardio-metabolic health and immune signatures in old individuals using daily chores (salat) as an intervention: a randomized crossover study in a little-studied population. *Frontiers in Public Health.* 2022;10:1009055. https://doi.org/10.3389/ fpubh.2022.1009055

18. Chokkhanchitchai, S., Tangarunsanti, T., Jaovisidha, S., Nantiruj, K., & Janwityanujit, S. The effect of religious practice on the prevalence of knee osteoarthritis. *Clinical Rheumatology.* 2010;29:39–44. https://doi.org/10.1007/ s10067-009-1295-8

19. Bukhari, A. *Attaining Health through Salah & Ablution.* Islamabad: Xlibris. 2015.

20. Osama, M. & Malik, R. J. Salat (Muslim prayer) as a therapeutic exercise. *Journal of Pakistan Medical Association.* 2019;69 (3):399–404.

21. Ijaz, S., Khalily, M. T., & Ahmed, I. Mindfulness in salah prayer and its association with mental health. *Journal of Religion and Health.* 2017;56:2297–307. https://doi.org/10 .1007/s10943-017-0413-1

22. Owens, J., Rassool, G. H., Bernstein, J., Latif, S., & Aboul-Enein, B. H. Interventions using the Qur'an to promote mental health: a systematic

scoping review. *Journal of Mental Health.* 2023;32(4):842–62. https://doi.org/10 .1080/09638237.2023.2232449

23. Denny, F. M. The meaning of "Ummah" in the Qur'ān. *History of Religions.* 1975;15(1):34–70. https://doi.org/10 .1086/462733

24. Pramesona, B. A. & Taneepanichskul, S. The effect of religious intervention on depressive symptoms and quality of life among Indonesian elderly in nursing homes: a quasi-experimental study. *Clinical Interventions in Aging.* 2018;13:473–83. https://doi.org/10.2147/ CIA.S162946

25. Toghyani, M., Kajbaf, M. B., & Ghamarani, A. Adherence to Islamic lifestyle as a cost-effective treatment for depression. *Mental Health, Religion & Culture.* 2018;21(8):797–809. https://doi .org/10.1080/13674676.2018.1551342

26. Rassool, G. H. The crescent and Islam: healing, nursing and the spiritual dimension. Some considerations towards an understanding of the Islamic perspectives on caring. *JAN.* 2000;32 (6):1476–84. https://doi.org/10.1046/j .1365-2648.2000.01614.x

27. Sabry, W. M. & Vohra, A. Role of Islam in the management of psychiatric disorders. *Indian Journal of Psychiatry.* 2013;55(Suppl 2):S205–14. https://doi .org/10.4103/0019-5545.105534

28. Koenig, H. G. Research on religion, spirituality, and mental health: a review. *Canadian Journal of Psychiatry.* 2009;54 (5):283–91. https://doi.org/10.1177/ 070674370905400502

29. Koenig, H. G., King, D. E., & Carson, V. B. *Handbook of Religion and Health.* 2nd ed. Oxford: Oxford University Press. 2012.

30. Koenig, H. G., Zaben, F. A., & Khalifa, D. A. Religion, spirituality and mental health in the West and the Middle East. *Asian Journal of Psychiatry.* 2012;5(2):180–82. https://doi.org/10.1016/j.ajp.2012.04.004

31. Attum, B., Hafiz, S., Malik, A., & Shamoon, Z. *Cultural Competence in the Care of Muslim Patients and Their Families.* In: StatPearls [online]. Treasure Island, FL: StatPearls Publishing. 2023. Available from: www.ncbi.nlm.nih.gov/ books/NBK499933/

32. Ezenkwele, U. A. & Roodsari, G. S. Cultural competencies in emergency medicine: caring for Muslim-American patients from the Middle East. *Journal of Emergency Medicine.* 2013;45(2):168–74. https://doi .org/10.1016/j.jemermed.2012.11.077

33. Hodge, D. R. Social work and the house of Islam: orienting practitioners to the beliefs and values of Muslims in the United States. *Social Work.* 2005;50:162–73. https://doi.org/10.1093/ sw/50.2.162

34. Halligan, P. Caring for patients of Islamic denomination: critical care nurses' experiences in Saudi Arabia. *Journal of Clinical Nursing.* 2006;15(12):1565–73. https://doi.org/10.1111/j.1365-2702.2005 .01525.x

35. Shaafi, S. & Kulkarni, H. Long-term practice of salat prevents Alzheimer's disease in humans: original study. *Alzheimer's & Dementia.* 2012;8 (4S:15):559. https://doi.org/10.1016/j.jalz .2012.05.1507

36. Antonovsky, A. *Health, Stress, and Coping.* 1st ed. San Francisco: Jossey-bass. 1979.

37. Antonovsky, A. *Unraveling the Mystery of Health: How People Manage Stress and Stay Well.* San Francisco: Jossey-Bass. 1987.

38. Antonovsky, A. The salutogenic model as a theory to guide health promotion. *Health Promotion International.* 1996;11 (1):11–18. https://doi.org/10.1093/ heapro/11.1.11

39. Eriksson, M. & Lindström, B. Validity of Antonovsky's sense of coherence scale: a systematic review. *Journal of Epidemiology and Community Health.* 2005;59(6):460–66. https://doi.org/10 .1136/jech.2003.018085

40. Lindström, B. & Eriksson, M. Salutogenesis. *Journal of Epidemiology and Community Health.* 2005;59 (6):440–42. https://doi.org/10.1136/jech .2005.034777

Perceptions of Health Behaviors and Illness in Muslims

G. Hussein Rassool

Introduction

"Bismillah Ar'Rahman Ar'Rahim." This statement, translated to "in the name of Allah, the most gracious, the most Merciful," is the opening words of the Qur'an that are frequently invoked by Muslims in health and sickness behaviors. The increased visibility of Muslim populations suggests the need for health care professionals to gain a better understanding of how the Islamic faith influences health-related perceptions and health care-seeking behaviors. Muslims are not a homogeneous community even though they may hold Islamic beliefs, cultural practices, institutions, and Islamic worldviews in common. This often proves challenging to health care professionals who are oriented toward a Eurocentric or Orientalist approach. However, there is some evidence to suggest there is increased recognition and understanding of health care professionals in the importance of religious and cultural practices in addressing the needs of Muslims [1]. In this chapter, the focus is on the examination of the perceptions of health behaviors and illness in Muslims that will assist health care professionals in delivering appropriate care in a culturally sensitive manner.

Health Beliefs, Health, and Illness Behaviors

Health belief systems are common in the worldview of most cultures "to explain the etiology of illness, the therapeutic interventions and who should be involved in the process (healthcare providers)" [2 p. 68]. Part of the dimension of health beliefs is the Islamic worldview (*Tasawur* or *Ru'yah al-Islam li al-Wujud*) which is based on the Qur'an and Sunnah. Akhmetova defined worldview as "a collection of positions, attitudes, values, stories and expectations about the world around us, which inform our every thought and action" [3]. This means that worldview is a subjective way of thinking and having a vision about and interacting with our world. Rassool suggested that the "Islamic worldview, based principally on a system of values and principles, derived from the Qur'an, is identical to the Qur'anic worldview. An Islamic worldview is related to both the seen world and the unseen world" [4 p. 7]. This ethical and monotheistic worldview stems from the fundamental belief in the unicity of God (*Tawhīd*). In addition to the *Tawhīdic* dimension, there is also an ethical (moral, or *akhlāq*) dimension of the Islamic worldview. An individual's perception and understanding of concepts such as "health," "illness," or "disease" arise from a complex interaction between personal experiences, a range of sociocultural factors, and religion [5]. These health beliefs are embedded with indigenous lay beliefs or cultural folktales. It is maintained that "ordinary people develop explanatory theories to account for their bodily circumstances" [6 p. 142]. Health beliefs may dictate privacy concerns; nutrition; sex in health consultations; modesty; personal hygiene; religious practices such as prayer; how health care information is desired and disseminated; sex and family roles in aspects of consent and confidentiality; processes for decision making; and how the care and interventions are managed. When providing care to Muslim patients, it is important to understand the effect the Islamic faith has on the provision and delivery of health care.

The Islamic Framework of Health

The Islamic notion of health is viewed in a holistic "whole person" approach and is established in the Qur'an and the Sunnah. *Ash-Shaafee* is one of the names of Allah, which has the meaning of "the One who cures."

The Qur'an is not only guidance for the whole of mankind but is a spiritual healing for all types of diseases. Allah mentions in the Qur'an, "*And when I am ill, it is He who cures me*" (Q Ash-Shu'ara 26:80). From an Islamic perspective, health is viewed as one of the greatest blessings that God has bestowed on humankind. The Prophet (PBUH) states, "There are two blessings which many people lose: [They are] Health and free time for doing good" [7]. In Muslim communities the influence of religion on shaping individual perception of health and illness behavior is often quite significant. It is stated that "Muslims believe that cure comes solely from Allah. Even if this is practically in the form of a health professional, it is still ultimately achieved through prayers and the powers of Allah" [8 p. 61]. Trials and tribulations are a part of life and a test from Allah. Allah says in the Qur'an, "*And We will surely test you with something of fear and hunger and a loss of wealth, lives, and fruits but give good tidings to the patient*" (Q Al-Baqarah 2:155). In the exegesis of Ibn Kathir [9], the above verse explains that Allah tests and tries us. Allah tests people with the afflictions of fear and hunger, the loss of wealth, and the loss of friends, relatives, and loved ones.

The health of Muslims is of paramount importance as being healthy means that they can adhere to Islamic practices and worship Allah. The Qur'an considers *Iman* (faith in Allah) as the foremost necessity for physical, spiritual, and mental health and stability. Stacey stated that "to fulfill the obligations of three of the five pillars of Islam requires that Muslims be of sound health and fitness. The daily performance of five prayers is in itself a form of exercise, its prescribed movements involve all the muscles and joints of the body, and concentration in prayer relieves mental stress. Good health is necessary if one intends to fast the month of *Ramadan* [fasting], and the performance of the *Hajj* (or pilgrimage to Mecca) is an arduous task that requires many days of hard physical effort" [6]. The health beliefs of Muslims, which are governed by the traditional Islamic value system and exemplified in the lifestyle of Prophet Muhammad (PBUH), can be used to justify engaging in positive health behaviors – that is, "enjoining what is good and forbidding what is wrong." Shayk-ul-Islam Ibn Taymiyyah stated that "enjoining right and forbidding wrong is done sometimes with the heart, sometimes with the tongue, and sometimes with the hand (for example, physical force). As for practicing it with the heart, it is obligatory upon everyone in every time and situation since its practice brings no hardship" [10]. In relation to health, enjoining right means doing the right thing through the process of a balanced diet, exercise, prayers adhering to the pillars of Islam and the principles of faith, and forbidding wrong by avoiding all forbidden (*haram*) behaviors and practices [10].

Preventive health behaviors of Muslims include personal hygiene and dental health, nutrition such as the restriction on eating specific ingredients (e.g., pork and its by-products), sexual health, avoidance of addictive habits such as alcohol and drug use (including tobacco and *shisha* smoking), avoidance of the overconsumption of food, exercise and physical activity, and spiritual development. Health in Islam is built on a wellness framework that aims to create individuals and a community that preserves and maintains their health through the guidance of the Qur'an and the Sunnah. This is in accordance with the salutogenic approach, focusing on factors that enhance positive health and well-being [11].

Perception of Health and Illness of the Muslim

Illness or wellness for an individual is a subjective interpretation that is viewed from that individual's worldview. In Islam, illness has three possible meanings: "a natural occurrence," "punishment of sin," or "a test of the believer's patience and gratitude" [12]. Muslims' health beliefs include beliefs to explain what causes illness, how it can be cured or treated (medical or religious therapies), and who should be involved in the process. A Muslim patient whose health belief is that their illness is a punishment from God for their past sins may not believe that biomedical care will help them. This is not a right way of thinking about illness; whether it is punishment or not, a Muslim is required to seek treatment.

A Muslim may believe that to achieve better health status the atonement for sins through prayers and doing good deeds, like giving to charity, must be performed [2]. There is extensive interest in understanding the attribution of health and illness based on the locus of control, which is the idea that an individual tends to understand events as controllable (an internal locus of control) or uncontrollable (an external locus of control). Health locus of control is defined as "a person's beliefs regarding where control over his/her health lies" [13 p. 534].

The term ascribed to the third force of health control is the spiritual health locus of control and the God locus of health control [13, 14, 15]. In Islam there is the belief in the Divine decree (*Qadar*), the sixth Islamic article of faith and human free will, and the use of both internal and external loci of control. Based on the above premises, the reliance solely on an internal locus of control "may not be congruent with many Muslims' belief in the power of external forces like God and the supernatural (e.g., angels, *Jinn*) in influencing their lives" [16 p. 100].

Having absolute trust in Allah (*Al-Tawakkul Alláh*) is a fundamental part of Muslim beliefs. That means trusting and being dependent on Allah. The following Hadith provides an example of having trust in and reliance on Allah (spiritual locus of control) and of making an effort to live in this world (internal locus of control). Anas ibn Malik reported that a man said, "O Messenger of Allah, should I tie my camel and trust in Allah, or should I leave her untied and trust in Allah?" The Messenger of Allah (PBUH) said, "Tie her and trust in Allah" [17]. The findings of a study by Aflakseir and Mohammad-Abadi showed that a God as the external locus of control was beneficial to mental health whereas an internal locus of control remained detrimental to mental health [18]. Notwithstanding the view that true faith requires total reliance on God (*Al-Tawakkul Alláh*), "recourse to an internal locus of control is not viewed as a weakness of belief, even if ill-health can also be seen as trials and tribulations by God meant for atonement and development in the purification of the soul" [13 p. 377].

Regardless of the cause, the sufferer must seek treatment, and many Hadiths encourage Muslims to seek medical treatment. Abu Hurairah narrated that the Prophet (PBUH) said, "There is no disease that Allah has created, except that He also has created its treatment" [19]. Muslims believe there is a cure provided for every illness and are encouraged to seek a cure through medical treatment. At the same time, a Muslim is always commanded to seek treatment and use medications that are derived from lawful (*halal*) origins. However, seeking treatment for ill health does not conflict with seeking help from Allah. Many Muslims do not seek help as they believe illness can and will purify the body. For this reason, many Muslims discard depression as an illness as it is seen to be related to a lack of faith [20]. From a religious perspective, Muslims understand recovery from any condition or deterioration as being only in the hands of Allah because He meant it to be that way. Abu Sa`id Al-Khudri and Abu Hurairah reported that the Prophet (PBUH) said, "No fatigue, nor disease, nor sorrow, nor sadness, nor hurt, nor distress befalls a Muslim, even if it were the prick he receives from a thorn, but that Allah expiates some of his sins for that" [21].

The findings from the research suggest some Muslims do not comply with medical treatments and with some types of medications. This may be due to religious injunctions that do not allow the use of particular medications or certain medical procedures [22]. For example, Muslims will not take some medications because many modern medications may contain unlawful pork derivates or alcohol which is strictly forbidden in the Islamic religion. This lack of adherence to treatment or medication regime may influence the treatment outcomes. There is a valuable insight into the health beliefs and Islamic values in a study conducted with Muslim patients living in the UK [23]. The findings showed that respect for the individual's dignity and privacy, community roles and importance, genuineness of provider, sex preference of the health care provider, modesty issues for men and women, language barriers, therapeutic touch, and the use of prayer and visitation of the sick for healing purposes were indicated as important [23]. Religious and cultural beliefs, such as the value placed on modesty and premarital virginity, contribute to reluctance to seek health care [24]. Following a study on help-seeking behavior and urinary incontinence in Muslim women, Sange found that many women felt it was religiously forbidden to seek help; however, many were unaware of the above statement [25].

Conclusion

The health beliefs and behaviors of Muslim patients have a significant effect on accessing and receiving health care. The beliefs that influence health behaviors in most Muslims are often carried in their culture's folktales and passed down over centuries through family health and healing practices. Understanding Muslim patients' beliefs about health practices, customs, and religious beliefs would be prime factors in the delivery of sensitive and culturally appropriate care to enhance positive health outcomes.

References

1. Hassan, S. M., Leavey, C., Rooney, J. S., & Puthussery, S. A qualitative study of healthcare professionals' experiences of providing maternity care for Muslim women in the UK. *BMC Pregnancy Childbirth*. 2020;20(1):400. https://doi.org/10.1186/s12884-020-03096-3

2. Rassool, G. H. *Health and Psychology: An Islamic Perspective*. Vol. 1. Beau Bassin-Rose Hill, MU: Islamic Psychology Publication (IPP), Amazon-Kindle. 2020.

3. Akhmetova, E. Week 3 worldviews. In: *Methodology of Scientific Research and Concept Formation (ITKI 6001)*. [MOOC]. Institute of Knowledge Integration. 2021 [Accessed March 23, 2023]. Available from: http://ikiacademy .org

4. Rassool, G. H. *Islamic Psychology: The Basics*. Oxford: Routledge. 2023.

5. Helman, C. G. *Culture, Health and Illness*. London: Arnold. 2001.

6. Stacey, A. Health in Islam (part 4 of 4): fitness and exercise. [online]. 2008 [Accessed March 23, 2023]. Available from: www.islamreligion.com/articles/ 1878/viewall/health-in-islam/

7. Sahih al-Bukhari. *Sahih al-Bukhari 6412*. In-book reference: Book 81, Hadith 1. Available from: https://sunnah.com/ bukhari:6412

8. Rassool, G. H. *Cultural Competence in Caring for Muslim Patients*. Basingstoke, UK: Palgrave Macmillan. 2014.

9. Kathir, I. Abualrub, J., Khitab, N., Khitab, H., Walker, A., Al-Jibali, M., & Ayoub, S., Trans. *Tafsir ibn Kathir*. Riyadh: Darussalam Publishers and Distributors. 2000.

10. Ibn Taymiyyah, S. U. I. *Al Amr Bil Ma'ruf wa Nahi 'Anil Munkar: Enjoining Right And Forbidding Wrong*. Sydney: International Centre for Islamic Studies. n.d.

11. Antonovsky, A. *Unravelling The Mystery of Health: How People Manage Stress and Stay Well*. San Francisco: Jossey-Bass Publishers. 1987.

12. Ibn Musa, A. *The Golden Epistle of Health (Resakat al-dhahabiya)*. Karachi: Peer Mohammed Ibrahim Trust. 1982.

13 Rassool, G. H. *Islamic Psychology: Human Behaviour and Experience from an Islamic Perspective*. Oxford: Routledge. 2021.

14. Debnam, K. J., Holt, C. L., Clark, E. M., Roth, D., Foushee, H. R., Crowther, M.,
et al. Spiritual health locus of control and health behaviors in African Americans. *American Journal of Health Behavior*. 2012;36(3):360–72. https://doi.org/10 .5993/AJHB.36.3.7

15. Meadows, R. J., Timiya, S., Nolan, T. S., & Paxton, R. J. Spiritual health locus of control and life satisfaction among African American breast cancer survivors. *Journal of Psychosocial Oncology*. 2020;38(3):343–57. https://doi .org/10.1080/07347332.2019.1692988

16. Amer, M. & Jalal, B. Individual psychotherapy/counseling: psychodynamic, cognitive behavioral and humanistic-experiential models. In: Ahmed, S. & Amer, M. M., eds. *Counseling Muslims: Handbook of Mental Health Issues and Intervention*. New York: Routledge. 2012. 87–117.

17. Tirmidhī. *Jami` at-Tirmidhi 2517*. In-book reference: Book 37, Hadith 103. Available from: https://sunnah.com/ tirmidhi:2517

18. Aflakseir, A. A. & Mohammad-Abadi, M. S. The role of health locus of control in predicting depression symptoms in a sample of Iranian older adults with chronic diseases. *Iranian Journal of Psychiatry*. 2016;11(2):82–86.

19. Sahih al-Bukhari. *Sahih al-Bukhari 5678*. In-book reference: Book 76, Hadith 1. Available from: https://sunnah.com/ bukhari:5678

20. Fonte, J. & Horton-Deutsch, S. Treating postpartum depression in immigrant Muslim women. *Journal of American Psychiatric Nurses Association*. 2005;11 (1):39–44. https://doi.org/10.1177/ 1078390305276494

21. Sahih al-Bukhari. *Sahih al-Bukhari 5642*. In-book reference: Book 75, Hadith 2. Available from: https://sunnah.com/ bukhari:5641

22. American Academy of Ophthalmology. Could religious beliefs affect compliance with ocular treatment? [online]. Science Daily. 2008 [Accessed March 24, 2023]. Available from: www.sciencedaily.com/ releases/2008/11/081109074608.htm

23. Cortis, J. D. Perceptions and experiences with nursing care: a study of Pakistani (Urdu) communities in the United Kingdom. *Journal of Transcultural Nursing.* 2000;11(2):111–18. https://doi.org/10.1177/104365960001100205

24. Matin, M. & LeBaron, S. Attitudes towards cervical cancer screening among Muslim women: A pilot study. *Women and Health.* 2004;39(3):63–77. https://doi.org/10.1300/j013v39n03_05

25. Sange, C. I am not being awkward: a hermeneutic phenomenological study on the perceptions of South Asian Muslim women and urinary incontinence. Unpublished PhD thesis. Lancashire, UK: University of Central Lancashire. 2009.

Social Justice, Human Rights, and Equality: An Islamic Perspective

Chapter 6

Huny Mohamed Amin Bakry, Eman Hassan Waly

Introduction

Healthy growth and progress of society require the integration of both social justice and development. Social justice is a necessity to meet the basic needs of the human being. The Holy Qur'an is considered the code of ethics for all Muslims. Several Qur'anic verses point out the different practices that support social justice and equality not only among Muslims but for every human being. This chapter explores social justice, human rights, and equality from the Holy Qur'anic perspective.

Definition of Social Justice

Social justice means everyone deserves equal basic needs or equal economic, political, and social rights or opportunities [1]. Social justice is one of the essential aspects of justice. Justice in Islam means "upholding the rights due to others or giving what is due to the person to whom it is due" [2]. All forms of justice among humankind including interpersonal, economic, or political interactions are considered social justice. *Qist* (fairness) is a Qur'anic term that describes social justice as a sense of equality and fairness in the distribution of resources, ensuring all individuals in society receive a fair share [3]. The Holy Qur'an encourages all people to follow justice and fairness in all activities of life:

> *O believers! Stand firm for justice as witnesses for Allah even if it is against yourselves, your parents, or close relatives. Be they rich or poor, Allah is best to ensure their interests. So do not let your desires cause you to deviate "from justice." If you distort the testimony or refuse to give it, then "know that" Allah is certainly All-Aware of what you do.*
>
> (Q An-Nisa 4:135)

Why We Should Apply Justice

The Holy Qur'an states, "*And the heaven, He has raised it high and he has set the balance*" (Q Ar-Rahman 55:7). This means that Allah has raised balance and justice since the beginning of the creation of the universe. The Just (*Al-Adl*) is one of Allah's Divine Names. The Holy Qur'an states, "*and (remember) when your Lord (Allah) said to the angels: Verily I am going to place mankind (Khalifah) generations after generations on earth*" (Q Al-Baqarah 2:79). Allah tells humankind that they are his *Khalifah* (custodian) on earth by emulating Allah's Divine Names. This task enables Allah's believers to embody the meanings of his Divine Names including justice and the promotion of virtues to the extent that is humanly possible [4].

Allah considers standing for justice as a fundamental characteristic of Him and the believers who know Him and feel his Grandeur. The Holy Qur'an states, "*Allah bears witness that la ilaha illa huwa (none has the right to be worshipped but he), the angels and those having knowledge (also give this witness); He always maintains his creation in justice*" (Q Al 'Imran 3:18). It also says, "*O you believe! Stand out firmly for justice, as witnesses to Allah, even though against yourselves, your parents, or your kin*" (Q An-Nisa 4:135). Moreover, Muslims are obligated to proactively participate in addressing any observed injustice and unfairness, "*enjoining good and forbidding evil*" (Q Al 'Imran 3:110; At-Tawbah 9:71).

Islam confirms that the elimination of injustice or oppression is an obligation. This obligation is on individual and community levels to establish a healthy society. According to the morals and ethics of Islam, it is forbidden to mention the faults of others in public except in the case of oppression. "*Allah does not like that evil to be uttered in public except by one who has been wronged, and Allah is Ever All-Hearer, All-Knower*" (Q An-Nisa 4:148).

Basic Elements of Social Justice in Islam

Social justice in Islam has three basic elements [5]. The first element is "freedom of conscience" which can be achieved by believing that the only superior authority upon human beings is Allah. The Holy Qur'an says, "*Say: None can protect me from Allah's punishment (If I were to disobey Him), nor can I find refuge except in Him*" (Q Al-Jinn 72:22). In other words, the fear of Allah gives an individual the strength to apply and promote justice. Allah set laws to ensure social justice and equality among humankind: "*O mankind; Be dutiful to your Lord, who created you from a single person (Adam) and from him (Adam), he created his wife (Hawwa), and from the both he created many men and women; and fear Allah through whom you demand (your mutual rights) and (do not cut the relations) the wombs (kinship). Surely, Allah is Ever an All-Watcher over you*" (Q An-Nisa 4:1).

The second element of social justice is **complete equality** to preserve human dignity for every human being, ensuring that only morals favor the individual rather than the class, biological sex, race, or color. Allah says, "*O mankind; we have created you from a male and a female and made you into nations and tribes, that you may know one another. Verily the most honorable of you with Allah is that who has At-Taqwa (piety). Verily, Allah is All-Knowing, All-Aware*" (Q Al-Hujuraat 49:13).

Social interdependence is the third essential element of social justice. It makes individuals responsible towards their community by sharing common goals and makes them influenced by their own and others' actions. These actions share in covering the basic requirements of disadvantaged individuals and providing emotional sympathy. The Holy Qur'an states, "*By no means shall you attain Al-Birr (piety, righteousness) unless you spend of that which you love; and whatever of good you spend, Allah knows it well*" (Q Al 'Imran 3:92).

Equitable Distribution of Wealth

Islam considers the unequal distribution of wealth among human beings as a natural thing; however, it does not welcome wide discrepancies. It encourages fairness in the distribution of economic resources or goods to all individuals in the community to narrow the wide gap between the rich and poor. This principle can be achieved through charity (zakat), which is an obligation on all sane adult Muslims who possess the *Nisab* (a minimum amount of wealth held for a year).

Zakat is manifested in The Holy Qur'an in many verses: "*And Perform As-Salat (the prayers) and give Zakat*" (Q Al-Baqarah 2:43, 2:83, 2:110; An-Nisa 4:77; At-Tawbah 9:103; an-Nur 24:56; Al-Muzzammil 73:20). Muslims should pay 2.5% of their assets to the poor, to those in bondage (slaves, captives, or debtors), and to others. "*Al-Sadaqat (voluntary charity) are only for the poor and those were employed to collect funds, those who have been inclined to Islam, and to free captives and debtors*" (Q At-Tawbah 9:60).

The Holy Qur'an provides several passages for the donation of voluntary charity (*Sadaqah*) confirming its great reward in the world and the hereafter: "*If you disclose your Sadaqat, it is well; but if you conceal them and give them to the poor, that is better for you, Allah will expiate you some of your sins. And Allah is Well-Acquainted with what you do*" (Q Al-Baqarah 2:271).

The Holy Qur'an mentions several measures other than zakat and *Sadaqah* in numerous verses as laws of inheritance, bequests, monetary atonement, and the prohibition of acquisition or hoarding of wealth that ensure social justice (Q An-Nisa 4:11–12, 4:176; Al-Baqarah 2:80; At-Tawbah 9:34–35).

Provision of Social Security and Protecting the Weak or Needy Individuals

The support of **orphans** is the responsibility of every Muslim. The Holy Qur'an states, "*Therefore, do not treat the orphan with oppression*" (Q Ad-Dhuha 93:9). Allah shows strict instructions in the Holy Qur'an emphasizing the health promotion of these vulnerable members of society through all means of physical, psychological, and monetary security. Protection of orphans' rights is mentioned more than twenty times in the Qur'an in different verses (Q Al-Baqarah 2:220; An-Nisa 4:2, 4:10, 4:127; Al-Isra' 17:34).

At the beginning of Islam during the sixth century, Islam prohibited the maltreatment of **enslaved people** and promoted the concept of emancipation. Islam accentuates that Allah created humankind free and that slavery is an assault on human freedom. Moreover, it encouraged freeing enslaved people by making it a way for the expiation of some kinds of sins. This is manifested in many Qur'anic verses. For instance, "*Allah will not punish you for what is unintended in your oaths, but He will punish you for your deliberate oaths; for their expiation feed ten Masakeen (poor people), on a scale of average of that with which you feed your own families, or clothe them, or free a slave*" (Q Al-Ma'idah 5:89). This verse directs the Muslims to provide weak, vulnerable groups with food, clothing, and financial support as community-based strategies to overcome their problems.

Islam also protects the rights of **captives** and sets rules that regulate their treatment. The Holy Qur'an states, after the end of a battle "*bind a bond firmly (take the enemies as captives). Thereafter, either Manna (for generosity) or Feda (redemption or ransom), until the war lays down its burden*" (Q Muhammad 47:4). *Manna* is regarded as the release of a captive without charge, and *Feda,* or redemption, is the release of a captive in exchange for money or service. Moreover, in another verse, the Holy Qur'an describes the Muslims who share food with the poor, orphans, and captives to be righteous: "*And they (pious or righteous) give the food, despite of their love for it, to the poor, orphan, and captive*" (Q Al-Insaan 76:8).

Regarding disabled individuals, Islam ensured showing respect and dignity to them. Islam exempted mentally and physically disabled individuals from obligatory duties like praying, zakat, hajj, or participation in military service. Allah says, at the time of war "*no blame or sin is there upon the blind, nor is there blame or sin upon the lame, nor is there blame or sin upon the sick*" (Q Al-Fath 48:17). In addition, the Holy Qur'an emphasized that the rights of people with disabilities should be appreciated and venerated and stated not to harm them in the form of ridicule and contempt: "*O, you who believe, do not let a group scoff at another group (disabled one), it may be that the latter are better than the former, nor women scoff at other women, it may be that the latter are better than the former, nor defame one another, nor insult one another by nicknames, ... then such are unjust (wrongdoers)*" (Q Al-Hujuraat 49:11).

In addition, Islam guarantees the rights of laborers against the employers. Prophet Muhammad (PBUH) said, "*Pay the laborer (worker) his wages or rights before his/her sweat dries up*" [6]. The wage of the workers is a fundamental obligation of the employer. The Holy Qur'an says, "*O my people, Give full measure and weight in justice and do not deduce the value of things that are due to the people, and do not commit mischief in the land, causing corruption*" (Q Hud 11:85). The Qur'an also mentions, "*O, you who believe, do not eat up one another's property (money) unjustly (in any illegal way)*" (Q Al-Baqarah 2:188; An-Nisa 4:29).

Provision of Social Equality to All People

Racial Equality

Islam promotes that all people are equal regardless of race and color except for genuine piety. "O humanity! Indeed, We (refers to Allah) created you from a male and a female and made you into nations and tribes so that you may get to know one another. Surely the noblest of you in the sight of Allah is the most righteous among you" (Q Al-Hujuraat 49:13). This was supported by Prophetic Hadiths; the messenger of Allah, Muhammad (PBUH) said, "That there is no difference between Arab and non-Arab People and between white or black person, but except in piety" [7].

Biological Sex Equality

Equality and justice do not have the same meaning in Islam. Justice for women does not mean equality with men in all aspects. There are many aspects of equality between men and women in Islam. However, Islam differentiated between men and women to the extent corresponding with the nature of each based on biological differences. The Holy Qur'an states, "*The male is not like the female*" (Q Al 'Imran 3:36). Each biological sex has the characteristics that suit it, and it is assigned to what suits it: "*Allah does not require of any soul more than what it can afford*" (Q Al-Baqarah 2:286).

Aspects of Equality between Men and Women

Islamic equality between men and women in rights is mentioned in the Holy Qur'an: "*Women have rights similar to those of men equitably, although men have a degree of responsibility above them*" (Q Al-Baqarah 2:228). Furthermore, the Holy Qur'an emphasizes biological sex equality in social reform responsibility: "*The believers, both men and women, are guardians of one another. They encourage good and forbid evil"* (Q At-Tawbah 9:71). The Holy Qur'an states, *"And their Lord responded to them, 'Never will I allow to be lost the work of [any] worker among you, whether male or female; you are of one another'"* (Q Al 'Imran 3:195). The Holy Qur'an also states, *"But those who do good – whether male or female – and have faith will enter Paradise"* (Q An-Nisa 4:124). Allah's preference over the other regarding man and woman is based on good deeds and piety: *"Surely the most noble of you in the sight of Allah is the most righteous among you"* (Q Al-Hujuraat 49:13). On a moral level, Islamic equality between men and women is also clear in the Holy Qur'an: *"O Prophet! Tell the believing men to lower their gaze and guard their chastity"* (Q An-Nur 24:30), *"and tell the believing women to lower their gaze and guard their chastity"* (Q An-Nur 24:31).

Aspects of Difference between Men and Women

The biological differences between men and women led to differences in physical, emotional, and volitional capacities. Man is charged with the guardianship of the family to provide and protect. Islam honored women by commanding men to treat women in a good manner and to take care of them: *"Treat them fairly"* (Q An-Nisa 4:19); *"Men are the caretakers of women, as men have been provisioned by Allah over women and tasked with supporting them financially"* (Q An-Nisa 4:34). In addition, Islam forbids oppressing women or oppressing their material or moral rights: *"Believers! It is not permissible for you to inherit women against their will or mistreat them"* (Q An-Nisa 4:19). Differentiation in some devotional issues aims to take care of women and to protect them with an appreciation for their circumstances. There are some things in which women differ from men in terms of Islamic rulings. Fasting and prayers are exempted for menstruating women as stated in the Hadith: "The Prophet (PBUH) said: Isn't it that when she menstruates, she does not pray or fast" [8].

Equality among Muslims and Non-Muslims

The Holy Qur'an was the constitution of Muslims in dealing with their opponents in religion, so it established a general law that the messenger of Allah, Muhammad (PBUH), and fellow Muslims adhered to in accordance with the Qur'an, which states, *"Let there be no compulsion in religion"* (Q Al-Baqarah 2:256). Muslims can support poor people (both Muslims and non-Muslims) through *Sadaqat* as stated in the Qur'an: *"Alms is only for the poor and the needy, for those employed to administer it, for those whose hearts are attracted 'to the faith,' for 'freeing' slaves, for those in debt, for Allah's cause, and for 'needy' travelers. This is an obligation from Allah. And Allah is All-Knowing, All-Wise"* (Q At-Tawbah 9:60). The Holy Qur'an urges Muslims to deal kindly with non-Muslim people: *"Allah does not forbid you from dealing kindly and fairly with those who have neither fought nor driven you out of your homes. Surely Allah loves those who are fair"* (Q Al-Mumtahanah 60:8).

Conclusion

The concept of justice is comprehensive and includes equality between people in rights and duties and giving each person their right. Social Justice, equity, and equality are frequently cited terms in the Holy Qur'an that guide the daily life activities of Muslims and should be adhered to by every Muslim without discrimination regardless of race, color, religion, or sex. However, the superiority of any individual is based on their piety and righteousness. Social justice and equality are fundamentals for health for all. Social justice and equality in health care access and elimination of disparities will enforce a healthy world. To quote Hadith an-Nawawi, "Whosoever of you sees an evil action, let him change it with his hand; and if he is not able to do so, then with his tongue; and if he is not able to do so, then with his heart; and that is the weakest of faith" [9].

References

1. San Diego Foundation. What is social justice? [online]. 2016 [Accessed June 3, 2023]. Available from: www.sdfoundation.org/news-events/sdf-news/what-is-social-justice.

2. Khan, N. A sacred duty: Islam and social justice. [online]. Yaqeen Institute. 2020 [Accessed June 4, 2023]. Available from: https://yaqeeninstitute.org/read/paper/a-sacred-duty-islam-and-social-justice

3. Harvey, R. Justice and mercy on the scale. [online]. Renovatio. 2017. Available from: https://renovatio.zaytuna.edu/article/justice-and-mercy-on-the-scale/

4. Al-Ghazali, A. Al-Khisht, M. U., ed. *Al-Maqsad al-asna fī sharh asma' Allah al-husna*. Cairo: Maktabat al-Qur'an. 1984.

5. Qutb, S. Hardie, J. B. & Algar, H., trans. *Social Justice in Islam*. Oneonta, NY: Islamic Publications International. 2000.

6. Sunan Ibn Majah. *Sunan Ibn Majah 2443*. In-book reference: Book 16, Hadith 8. Available from: https://sunnah.com/ibnmajah:2443

7. International Islamic University Malaysia. The last sermon of Prophet Muhammad (PBUH). [online]. [Accessed July 4, 2023]. Available from: https://www.iium.edu.my/deed/articles/thelastsermon.html

8. Sahih al-Bukhari. *Sahih al-Bukhari 1951*. In-book reference: Book 30, Hadith 58. Available from: https://sunnah.com/bukhari:1951

9. An-Nawawi. *Hadith 34, 40 Hadith an-Nawawi*. Available from: https://sunnah.com/nawawi40:34

Public Health, Hygiene, and Islam

Howeida Hassan Abusalih, Husameldin Elsawi Khalafalla

Introduction

Islam, as a way of life, directs its followers in matters conducive to public health. This is achieved through messages contained in the Holy Qur'an and the teachings of Prophet Muhammad (PBUH) who stated, "Cleanliness in Islam is considered half [of Islamic] faith" [1]. For personal hygiene, Muslims are expected to keep their bodies clean, which is portrayed in some rituals that precede many actions, as in the case of praying. Muslims are also advised on personal hygiene regarding the care of nails, hair, and clothes. Additionally, Muslims are obliged to keep their environment clean and are prohibited from polluting running sources of water and public places [2].

Infectious diseases and epidemics are major public health concerns. Islamic teachings help mitigate their negative impact on societies. In the early times of Islam, the teachings in the Holy Qur'an and the guidance of the Prophet Muhammad (PBUH) advised Muslims on how to deal with these public health issues by giving instruction on personal hygiene and travel restrictions [3].

Public health aims to promote and protect the health of people and the communities where they live. The teachings of Islam on personal and environmental hygiene as well as on how to deal with communicable diseases and epidemics are still relevant today. Hand washing, travel restrictions, and quarantine are considered important contributors to the control of a pandemic. Muslims thus hold a strong belief that the teachings of Islam that encompass many aspects of our lives are relevant to infection control and prevention [4].

In this chapter, Islamic teachings and practices pertaining to public health and hygiene as well as guidelines on how to deal with infectious disease and epidemics are outlined in accordance with contemporary evidence-based practices and guidelines.

Types of Hygiene

Hygiene can be divided into personal hygiene represented by the cleanliness of the body and clothes and public hygiene represented by environmental hygiene.

Personal Hygiene

Personal hygiene is an essential component of *ibadah* (worship) for obtaining Allah's favor [5]. Bodily cleanliness is advised in general and in the acts of worship in Islam that are preceded by procedures involving cleanliness of the body and clothes and is considered fundamental to the Islamic faith. The Prophet Muhammad (PBUH) declared that "cleanliness is half faith or the twin-half of faith," reported by Abu Malik at-Ash'ari [1]. Maintaining proper personal hygiene and washing one's body and hair with soap and water regularly help to prevent or control many infectious diseases [6]. Personal hygiene in Islam can be divided into three categories:

1. Purification from impurity (i.e., to attain purity or cleanliness, by taking a bath [*ghusl*] or performing ablution [*wudu*] in states in which a bath or ablution is necessary or desirable according to Islamic law) [1]
2. Cleansing one's body, dress, or place from impurity or filth [1]
3. Removing the dirt that collects in various parts of the body, such as the trimming of nails or excess unwanted hairs [1]
4. Adding perfumes [1]

Purification from Impurity
Ablution (*wudu*)

Ablution (*wudu*) is an act that must be performed before engaging in worship activities, especially the prayers or circumambulating the Ka'bah, Islam's holiest site in Mecca. As stated in the Holy Qur'an: "*O believers! When you rise up for prayer, wash your faces and your hands up to the elbows, wipe your heads, and wash your feet to the ankles*" (Q Al-Ma'idah 5:6). Muslims also conduct ablution before reading the Holy Qur'an and before going to bed. Performing ablution (*wudu*) in Islam is thought to be one of the most purifying ways to clean parts of the body. To do a full ablution, one must wash their face, including their mouth and nose up to their throats, their two hands up to their elbows, their head, their ears, their neck, and their feet up to their ankles. The Prophet Muhammad (PBUH) said, "If any Muslim performs ablution well then stands and prays two Rak'ahs [iterations of prostrations and supplications during praying] while focused on them with his heart and his face, Paradise is guaranteed for him" [7]. The Prophet Muhammad (PBUH) also said, "Whenever you go to bed, perform ablution like that for the prayer, and lie on your right side" [8].

One of the most crucial precautions to take to avoid getting ill and infecting others is practicing good hand hygiene by doing hand washing through *wudu* five times a day before prayers, thereby helping to reduce the risk of potential pathogens and potentially preventing infections [9]. The Prophet Muhammad (PBUH) said, "He who goes to sleep with his hands smelling of grease and suffers something evil in consequence shall have no one but himself to blame" [10]. Good hand hygiene is one of the most efficient strategies to stop the transmission of infectious diseases, leading to lower morbidity and mortality [11].

Islamic Shower and Bathing

Islamic shower, *Ghusl,* or *Ghusl-Janabat,* is a ritual of covering the whole body with water and is often performed in certain steps the way that the Prophet Muhammad (PBUH) performed it. "*If you are in a state of janaba* (ritual impurity), *purify yourself* (bathe your whole body)" (Q Al-Ma'idah 5:6). This ritual bathing precedes certain occasions, some of which are mandatory as in the case of burial. Muslims are required to perform a *ghusl* after sexual intercourse and at the end of a menstrual cycle [12].

Muslims are also required to bathe before participating in the weekly Friday prayer, for the two-yearly Islamic feasting holidays (*Eid Al-Fitr* and *Eid Al-Adha*), when making Pilgrimage or *Umra* (voluntary pilgrimage), whenever they feel unclean, and for other social gathering occasions. The Prophet Muhammad (PBUH) is reported to have said, "To take a bath on Friday is a duty of every pubescent Muslim" [13]. He also said the following:

> Whoever takes a bath on a Friday and does it well, and purifies himself and does it well, and puts on his best clothes, and puts on whatever Allah decrees for him of the perfume of his family, then comes to the mosque and does not engage in idle talk or separate (pushing between) two people; he will be forgiven for (his sins) between that day and the previous Friday. [14]

Cutting Nails, Removing Unnecessary Body Hair, Wearing Clean Clothes, and Adding Perfumes

Certain infections can spread via contaminated dirt and potential pathogens that parts of the body such as fingernails can contain. Fingernails should be kept short and washed regularly with soap and water on the undersides. Chewing or biting your nails should be avoided, as well as cutting cuticles [15]. Cutting and trimming nails are from *Sunnah al-Fitrah* (the natural state and act of cleanliness according to the Prophet [PBUH]). The Prophet Muhammad (PBUH) said, "Five practices are characteristic of the *fitra*: circumcision, shaving the pubic hair, cutting the moustache short, clipping the nails, and removing the hair of the armpits" [16]. Also, Sunan an-Nasa'i stated that to keep one's personal hygiene, the Prophet recommended regular practice of cutting finger and toenails and removing pubic and armpit hair [17], thereby reducing odor-producing microbes. It is said that the Prophet (PBUH) was known to love good smells, and he stated, "Perfume have been made dear to me, and my comfort has been provided in prayer" [18].

Coughing and Sneezing

As highlighted earlier, one of the most important aspects of hygiene in Islam is the consistency of cleanliness, which is necessary for personal hygiene to prevent a person from certain infectious diseases. Islam contains explicit prohibitions against publicly sneezing and coughing. When sneezing, the followers of Prophet Muhammad (PBUH) were commanded to conceal their faces [19]. The spread of airborne bacteria and viruses is the most apparent consequence of sneezing and coughing without covering the mouth.

Environmental Hygiene

Islam endeavors to protect the environment and keep it clean. The Prophet Muhammad (PBUH) warned, "Guard against the three things which cause curse (i.e.) defecating at the watering places, on the roadbeds and in the shades." [20]. The Prophet Muhammad (PBUH) forbade anyone to urinate or defecate in stagnant water [21].

Social Distancing, Isolation, and Quarantine

Muslims are advised to avoid contact with infected people, which the Prophet Muhammad (PBUH) was reported to advise [22]. According to Sahih Muslim, a man who was known to suffer from leprosy wanted to pledge his allegiance to Islam to the Prophet Muhammad (PBUH) by shaking hands with the Prophet and his companions.

The Prophet politely declined by informing the man with leprosy, "We have accepted your allegiance, so you may go" [22].

In cases of epidemics, it was reported that the Prophet (PBUH) ordered his followers to stay away from areas with diseases and, if somebody is already in that area, not to leave it by saying, "If you hear that there is a plague in a land, do not enter it; and if it (plague) visits a land while you are therein, do not go out of it" [3].

The practices of isolation, quarantine, the avoidance of close contact with infected people, and the control of movement to and from an area are practices that remain useful in containing infectious diseases in general, and particularly in light of the recent COVID-19 pandemic. Regarding the effectiveness of social distancing, Matrajt and Leung observed that even in the modest forms of social distancing, most new cases, hospitalizations, and fatalities were avoided when social distancing strategies were in place, and a rebound of cases was observed when they were lifted [23]. Wang et al. concluded that even a modest implementation of social distancing can provide valuable time for the health care system to recover and control the epidemic. They also highlighted the importance of the simultaneous implementation of other measures such as testing and contact tracing [24].

Conclusion

The teachings of Islam are an important contribution to achieving the public health goal of protecting the health of people and communities. These teachings contained in the Holy Qur'an and Prophetic instruction guided followers in pursuing good personal and environmental hygiene as well as in taking precautions to deal with infectious diseases and epidemics. These teachings are useful and relevant in controlling epidemics and infectious diseases and are in line with current evidence-based recommendations.

References

1. Sahih Muslim. *Sahih Muslim 223*. In-book reference: Book 2, Hadith 1. Available from: https://sunnah.com/muslim:223

2. Aboul-Enein, B. H. "The earth is your mosque": narrative perspectives of environmental health and education in the Holy Quran. *Journal of Environmental Studies and Sciences.* 2017;8:22–31. https://doi.org/10.1007/s13412-017-0444-7

3. Sahih al-Bukhari. *Sahih al-Bukhari 5728*. In-book reference: Book 76, Hadith 43. Available from: https://sunnah.com/bukhari:5728

4. Mutalib, L. A., Ismail, W. A. F. W., Baharuddin, A. S., Mohamed, M. F., Abd Murad, A. H., et al. Scientific exegesis of al-quran and its relevance in dealing with contemporary issues: an appraisal on the book of 'al-jawahir fi tafsir al-quran al-karim. *International Journal of Recent Technology and Engineering.* 2019;8(2-S11):575–81. https://doi.org/10.35940/ijrte.b1089.0982s1119

5. Omar, S. H. S., Mohd Safri, A., Musa, R., Zin, A. D. M., Wahid, N. A., Fazli, A., et al. A means of attaining Ma`Rifah Allah according to Al-Qushayri. *International Journal of Civil Engineering and Technology.* 2018:9(13):194–98.

6. Centers for Disease Control and Prevention. Water, sanitation, and environmentally related hygiene (WASH). [online]. 2022 [Accessed April 13, 2023]. Available from: www.cdc.gov/hygiene/about/index.html

7. Sahih Muslim. *Sahih Muslim 234a*. In-book reference: Book 2, Hadith 20. Available from: https://sunnah.com/muslim:234a

8. Sahih al-Bukhari. *Sahih al-Bukhari 247.* In-book reference: Book 4, Hadith 113. Available from: https://sunnah.com/bukhari:247

9. Bajirova, M. Hygiene and health in Quran and science. *EC Gynecology SPI.* 2017;1: P44–55.

10. Sunan Ibn Majah. *Sunan Ibn Majah 1097.* In-book reference: Book 5, Hadith 295. Available from: https://sunnah.com/ibnmajah:1097

11. Allegranzi, B. & Pittet, D. Role of hand hygiene in healthcare-associated infection prevention. *Journal of Hospital Infection.* 2009;73:305–15. https://doi.org/10.1016/j.jhin.2009.04.019

12. Muwatta Malik. *Purity.* Book 2, Hadith 128. Available from: https://sunnah.com/urn/501280

13. Sahih al-Bukhari. *Sahih al-Bukhari 879.* In-book reference: Book 11, Hadith 4. Available from: https://sunnah.com/bukhari:879

14. Sunan Ibn Majah. *Sunan Ibn Majah 1097.* In-book reference: Book 5, Hadith 295. Available from: https://sunnah.com/ibnmajah:1097

15. Sahih al-Bukhari. *Sahih al-Bukhari 5890.* In-book reference: Book 77, Hadith 107. Available from: https://sunnah.com/bukhari:5890

16. Sunan an-Nasa'i. *Sunan an-Nasa'I 11.* In-book reference: Book 1, Hadith 11. Available from: https://sunnah.com/nasai:11

17. Ahl al-Hadith. Rulings and etiquette of sneezing in Islamic law. [online]. The Modern Comprehensive Library. 2023 [Accessed April 13, 2023]. Available from: https://al-maktaba.org/book/31616/49738#p3

18. Sunan an-Nasa'i. *Sunan an-Nasa'i 3939.* In-book reference: Book 36, Hadith 1. Available from: https://sunnah.com/nasai/36/1

19. Sahih Muslim. *Sahih Muslim 223.* In-book reference: Book 2, Hadith 1. Available from: https://sunnah.com/muslim:223

20. Bulugh al-Maram. *Bulugh al-Maram 92.* In-book reference: Book 1, Hadith 110. Available from: https://sunnah.com/bulugh:92

21. Sahih Muslim. *Sahih Muslim 281.* In-book reference: Book 2, Hadith 121. Available from: https://sunnah.com/muslim:281

22. Sahih Muslim. *Sahih Muslim 2231.* In-book reference: Book 39, Hadith 174. Available from: https://sunnah.com/muslim:2231

23. Matrajt, L. & Leung, T. Evaluating the effectiveness of social distancing interventions to delay or flatten the epidemic curve of coronavirus disease. *Emerging Infectious Diseases.* 2020;26 (8):1740–48. https://doi.org/10.3201/eid2608.201093

24. Wang, X., Pasco, R. F., Du, Z, Petty, M., Fox, S. J., Galvani, A. P., et al. Impact of social distancing measures on coronavirus disease healthcare demand, central Texas, USA. *Emerging Infectious Diseases.* 2020;26 (10):2361–69. https://doi.org/10.3201/eid2610.201702

Chapter 8

Foods of the Qur'anic Garden: An Islamic Perspective

Elizabeth Dodge

Introduction

Many religious and cultural health and food practices have roots in religious texts and beliefs [1–7], and these beliefs and practices can impact dietary and food choices as well as health [8–11]. For Muslims, the teachings of the Holy Qur'an provide spiritual and behavioral guidance. Because religiosity and cultural beliefs and practices influenced by religion can affect food and health behavior, it is imperative to understand and explore the guidance provided through religious teachings [12–16]. This chapter examines Qur'anic guidance on food, nutrition, and dietary practices. It also investigates the historical alignment of Qur'anic guidance with the Mediterranean diet (MedDiet), a dietary pattern that exhibits substantial overlap with the foodways and practices of Muslim populations in the Middle East and North Africa (MENA) [10, 17–19].

Qur'anic Food Guidance

Other literature has covered the specific Qur'anic passages and verses that govern food, dietary practices, and beliefs of the Muslim communities in detail [4, 9, 10, 13, 20–23]. For example, Khalid and Sediqi [3] noted 257 verses in the Holy Qur'an that address food and nutrition, while other verses contain words specific to disease (171 verses), eating (109 verses), and drinking (131 verses); additional verses describe food and dietary practices. Aboul-Enein [20] provided an analysis of 36 passages that detail the use of grains, fruits, and vegetables. One such Qur'anic verse is as follows: "*And it is He Who produced gardens, both trellised and untrellised, and date palms, and crops of different shape and taste (their fruits and their seeds) and olives, and pomegranates, similar (in kind) and different (in taste). Eat of the fruits when they ripen*" (Q Al-An'am 6:141). Another verse states: "*And when you said, O Moses! We cannot endure one kind of food. Therefore, pray to your Lord to produce for us what the earth grows, its herbs, its cucumbers, its wheat or garlic, lentils, and onions*" (Q Al-Baqarah 2:61). The consensus from the literature is that Qur'anic guidance, particularly as it relates to food items, provides direct reference to 19 plants, described in Latin name by Khalid et al. as: "*Alhagi maurorum, Allium cepa, Allium sativum, Brassica nigra, Cinamoumon camphor, Cucumis sativus, Cucurbita pepo, Ficus carica, Lens culinaris Medic, Musa sapientum, Ocimum basilicum, Olea europaea, Phoenix dactylifera, Punica granatum, Salvadora persica, Tamarix aphylla, Vitis vinifera, Zingiber officinale,* and *Ziziphus spina-christi*" [3]. The plant species listed above include legumes and lentils, alliums such as onion, leeks, and garlic, spices and herbs such as mustard, basil, and ginger, and fruits and vegetables such as bananas/plantains, figs, grapes, pomegranates, palm dates, pumpkins, cucumbers, sidr/jujube, and olives (including olive oil). Another article notes 23 Qur'anic passages mentioning a variety of foods including grains, seeds, herbage, fish and seafood, milk and dairy, and honey [10].

The Mediterranean Diet: Regional Variations and Global Adoption

The traditional MedDiet is thought to have been popularized by work completed by Ancel Keys in the 1950s [24] and has been described as a dietary pattern "followed by populations of olive tree-growing areas around the Mediterranean basin" [24], which, as pointed out by Obeid et al., would include countries such as "Albania, Algeria, Bosnia, Croatia, Cyprus, Egypt, France, Gibraltar, Greece, Israel, Italy, Lebanon, Libya, Morocco, Malta, Monaco, Montenegro, occupied Palestinian territory and Gaza strip, Slovenia, Spain, Syria, Turkey, and Tunisia" [25]. Researchers agree the wider geographic origin of the MedDiet, including countries in and around the Mediterranean basin, is reflective of the basis of the dietary pattern, with some regional differences [5, 26–28].

However, there has been recent criticism of the "MedDiet" that global consumers have learned about due to its positive health impacts [29–34] and that is rather a "Eurocentric" MedDiet that has been informed by limiting the populations historically assumed to consume this diet to the European Mediterranean. Indeed, much of the research related to the health benefits of the diet places a heavy emphasis on European Mediterranean dietary patterns [35, 36], often neglecting the more diverse and regionally oriented depictions of the MedDiet adhered to by many in non-European Mediterranean countries, including those in MENA [37]. Still, the basic principles of the MedDiet, the research on the health benefits of globally adapted Mediterranean dietary patterns, and the adoption of these principles and patterns by many proponents of health are prevalent in the literature [12–16].

Cultural Congruency of the Mediterranean Diet with Qur'anic Guidance

Despite the discussions regarding omissions of the complete origins of the MedDiet in the literature, the Mediterranean dietary pattern, taken as a whole and inclusive of countries in Europe, Northern Africa, and the Middle East, is largely culturally congruent with Qur'anic guidance. The MedDiet emphasizes whole grains, plant oils, fruits and vegetables, nuts, and legumes; suggests fish/poultry or egg and dairy/fermented dairy consumption up to two times a day; and recommends limited consumption of food products typical of the Western pattern diet such as red meat, butter, white/refined grains, and sweets [27, 38, 39]. Regarding the suggestion of red wine in Mediterranean food guidance, this should always have the caveat "when/as appropriate." In Islam, drinking alcohol is *haram* (forbidden) [40, 41], and additional considerations should be given to those who may suffer from alcohol use disorder [35, 38].

In addition to guidance on specific appropriate (*halal*) foods to include in the diet, the Holy Qur'an also offers guidance on acceptable food production, preparation, and storage techniques [3, 7, 20, 41–44]. Examples of such Qur'anic verses include: "*And do they not see that We drive water to parched soil (bare of herbage), and produce therewith crops, providing food for their cattle and themselves? Have they not the vision?*" (Q As-Sajdah 32:27) [43], "*Eat of their fruits when they come to fruition, and give (to the poor and the needy) the due thereof on harvest day. And do not be wasteful; indeed God does not love the wasteful"* (Q Al-An'am 6:141) [43], as well as *"And [We brought forth] an olive tree issuing from Mount Sinai which produces oil and [it is a] relish for those who eat"* (Q Al-Mu'minun 23:20) [20]. Additionally, the Prophetic guidance reflects upon the preparation of animal foods: "Verily Allah has enjoined goodness to everything; so when you kill, kill in a good way and when you slaughter, slaughter in a good way. So every one of you should sharpen his knife, and let the slaughtered animal die comfortably" [44, 45]. As it relates to viewing the tenets of the MedDiet through the lens of Qur'anic guidance, some authors also emphasize the importance of the concept of *tayyib* (wholesome) as it relates to food preparation and/or preservation [41, 42]. *Halal* and *tayyib* foods mirror the foundational components of the Mediterranean dietary pattern as *tayyib* can be related to the consumption of whole or minimally refined foods, particularly the plant-based foods discussed above [42, 43, 46–48]. In addition, *halal* and *tayyib* standards can also be applied to food preservation practices including sanitary preparation and packaging integrity of processed *halal* foods [46–48].

Conclusion

There is symmetry and cultural congruency around healthful dietary practices and health benefits conferred by specific foods mentioned in the Holy Qur'an and the majority of the components emphasized in the MedDiet (with exception to the consumption of alcohol, which is considered *haram*). This information can be used to tailor acceptable and healthful dietary patterns for those in Muslim communities. Further, the health benefits of the traditional dietary patterns of Mediterranean countries, including MENA regions, have served as the basis for dietary practice in those countries and have been widely adopted globally for health interventions.

References

1. Farouk, M. M., Regenstein, J. M., Pirie, M. R., Najm, R., Bekhit, A. E., & Knowles, S. O. Spiritual aspects of meat and nutritional security: perspectives and responsibilities of the Abrahamic faiths. *Food Research International.* 2015;76:882–95. https://doi.org/10.1016/j.foodres.2015.05.028

2. Bosire, E. N., Cele, L., Potelwa, X., Cho, A, & Mendenhall, E. God, church water and spirituality: perspectives on health and healing in Soweto, South Africa. *Global Public Health.* 2022;17(7):1172–85. https://doi.org/10.1080/17441692.2021.1919738

3. Khalid, S. M. N. & Sediqi, S. M. Improving nutritional and food security status in Muslim communities: integration of Qur'anic practices in development programs – a review. *International Journal of Nutrition Sciences.* 2018;3(2):65–72.

4. Ailin Qian. Delights in paradise: a comparative survey of heavenly food and drink in the Qur'an. In: Sebastian Günther & Todd Lawson, eds. *Roads to Paradise: Eschatology and Concepts of the Hereafter in Islam.* Vol. 1. Leiden: Brill. 2017. 251–70. https://doi.org/10.1163/9789004333154_012

5. Berry, E. M., Arnoni, Y., & Aviram, M. The Middle Eastern and biblical origins of the Mediterranean diet. *Public Health Nutrition.* 2011;14(12A):2288–95. https://doi.org/10.1017/s1368980011002539

6. Odukoya, O. O., Odediran, O., Rogers, C. R., Ogunsola, F., & Okuyemi, K. S. Barriers and facilitators of fruit and vegetable consumption among Nigerian adults in a faith-based setting: a pre-intervention qualitative inquiry. *Asian Pacific Journal of Cancer Prevention:*

APJCP. 2022;23(5):1505–11. https://doi .org/10.31557/apjcp.2022.23.5.1505

7. Roudsari, A. H., Vedadhir, A., Amiri, P., Kalantari, N., Omidvar, N., Eini-Zinab, H., et al. Psycho-socio-cultural determinants of food choice: a qualitative study on adults in social and cultural context of Iran. *Iranian Journal of Psychiatry.* 2017;12(4):241.

8. Truong, M., Paradies, Y., & Priest, N. Interventions to improve cultural competency in healthcare: a systematic review of reviews. *BMC Health Services Research.* 2014;14(1):1–7. https://doi.org/ 10.1186/1472-6963-14-99

9. Hibban, M. F. Living Qur'an and Sunnah as the foundation of a holistic healthy lifestyle. *International J. of Islamic and Complementary Medicine.* 2022;3 (2):49–56. https://doi.org/10.55116/ IJICM.V3I2.40

10. Aboul-Enein, B. H. Reflections of the Holy Qur'an and the Mediterranean diet: a culturally congruent approach to obesity? *Mediterranean Journal of Nutrition and Metabolism.* 2015;8(2):149–54. http://doi .org/10.3233/MNM-150041

11. Bouchareb, S., Chrifou, R., Bourik, Z., Nijpels, G., Hassanein, M., Westerman, M. J., et al. "I am my own doctor": a qualitative study of the perspectives and decision-making process of Muslims with diabetes on Ramadan fasting. *PLoS ONE.* 2022;17(3):e0263088. https://doi.org/10 .1371/journal.pone.0263088

12. Sheikh, B. Y. The role of prophetic medicine in the management of diabetes mellitus: a review of literature. *Journal of Taibah University Medical Sciences.* 2016;11(4):339–52. https://doi.org/10 .1016/j.jtumed.2015.12.002

13. Iqbal, A. S., Jan, M. T., Muflih, B. K., & Jaswir, I. The role of prophetic food in the prevention and cure of chronic diseases: a review of literature. *Malaysian Journal of Social Sciences and Humanities (MJSSH).* 2021;6(11):366–75. https://doi.org/10 .47405/mjssh.v6i11.1144

14. Basir, S. M., Shukri, N. A., Ghani, R. A., Ibrahim, M., Khattak, M. M., & Omar, M.

N. Assessment of prophetic foods consumption among lactating mothers: combining quantitative & qualitative approaches. *IIUM Medical Journal Malaysia.* 2018;17(1):181–85. http://doi .org/10.31436/imjm.v17i1.1015

15. Salarvand, S. & Pournia, Y. Perception of medical university members from nutritional health in the Qur'an. *Iranian Red Crescent Medical Journal.* 2014;16 (4):1–8. https://doi.org/10.5812/ircmj .10846

16. Green, J., Draper, A., & Dowler, E. Short cuts to safety: risk and "rules of thumb" in accounts of food choice. *Health, Risk & Society.* 2003;5(1):33–52. https://doi.org/ 10.1080/1369857031000065998

17. Farhangi, H., Ajilian, M., Saeidi, M., & Khodaei, G. H. Medicinal fruits in the holy Qur'an. *International Journal of Pediatrics.* 2014;2(3.2):89–102. http://dx .doi.org/10.22038/ijp.2014.3461

18. Sandhu, A. K., Islam, M., Edirisinghe, I., & Burton-Freeman, B. Phytochemical composition and health benefits of figs (fresh and dried): a review of literature from 2000 to 2022. *Nutrients.* 2023;15 (11):2623.1–27. https://doi.org/10.3390/ nu15112623

19. Heidari, M. R. Cardiovascular effects of olive, a Qur'anic fruit: a systematic review. *Journal of Islamic and Iranian Traditional Medicine.* 2016;7(1):21–30.

20. Aboul-Enein, B. H. "The Qur'anic garden": consumption of fruits, vegetables, and whole grains from an Islamic perspective. *International Journal of Multicultural & Multireligious Understanding.* 2017;4(4):53–63. http:// doi.org/10.18415/ijmmu.v4i4.78

21. Hussain, N. H., Hassan, K., & Akhir, N. M. Contemplating the Islamic garden and Malay traditional landscape from the Qur'an. *Asian Journal of Behavioural Studies.* 2018;3(13):46–53. https://doi.org/ 10.21834/ajbes.v3i13.142

22. Goje, D. K. Preventive prophetic medicine in foods and beverages: an analytic study. *Hamdard Islamicus.* 2021;44(3):87–104.

23. Kabiru, G. M. & Samarh, S. N. A. Preventive medicine in food and drink: an analytic study of the Islamic approach. *Review of International Geographical Education (RIGEO)*. 2021;11(8):2657–65.

24. Trichopoulou, A., Martínez-González, M. A., Tong, T. Y., Forouhi, N. G., Khandelwal, S., Prabhakaran, D., et al. Definitions and potential health benefits of the Mediterranean diet: views from experts around the world. *BMC medicine*. 2014;12(1):1–6. https://doi.org/10.1186/1741-7015-12-112

25. Obeid, C. A., Gubbels, J. S., Jaalouk, D., Kremers, S. P. J., & Oenema, A. Adherence to the Mediterranean diet among adults in Mediterranean countries: a systematic literature review. *European Journal of Nutrition*. 2022;61(7):3327–44. https://doi.org/10.1007/s00394-022-02885-0

26. Manios, Y., Detopoulou. V., Visioli. F., & Galli, C. Mediterranean diet as a nutrition education and dietary guide: misconceptions and the neglected role of locally consumed foods and wild green plants. In: Galli, C., Heinrich, M., & Muller, W. E., eds. *Local Mediterranean Food Plants and Nutraceuticals*. Berlin: Karger. 2006. 154–70. https://doi.org/10.1159/000095212

27. Sahyoun, N. R. & Sankavaram, K. Historical origins of the Mediterranean Diet, regional dietary profiles, and the development of the dietary guidelines. In: Romagnolo, D. & Selmin, O., eds. *Mediterranean Diet*. Totowa, NJ: Humana Press, 2016. 28–67.

28. Daou, T., Abi Kharma, J., Daccache, A., Bassil, M., Naja, F., & Rahi, B. Association between Lebanese Mediterranean diet and frailty in community-dwelling Lebanese older adults: a preliminary study. *Nutrients*. 2022;14(15):3084.1–15. https://doi.org/10.3390/nu14153084

29. Esposito, S., Gialluisi, A., Costanzo, S., Di Castelnuovo, A., Ruggiero, E., De Curtis, A., et al. Mediterranean diet and other dietary patterns in association with biological aging in the Moli-sani study cohort. *Clinical Nutrition*. 2022;41 (5):1025–33. https://doi.org/10.1016/j.clnu.2022.02.023

30. Georgoulis, M., Yiannakouris, N., Tenta, R., Fragopoulou, E., Kechribari, I., Lamprou, K., et al. A weight-loss Mediterranean diet/lifestyle intervention ameliorates inflammation and oxidative stress in patients with obstructive sleep apnea: results of the "MIMOSA" randomized clinical trial. *European Journal of Nutrition*. 2021;60 (7):3799–810. https://doi.org/10.1007/s00394-021-02552-w

31. Burch, J. & Thapa, B. How does a Mediterranean-style diet compare with a low-fat diet for the primary prevention of cardiovascular disease (CVD)? [online] Cochrane Clinical Answers. 2019 [Accessed April 5, 2023]. Available from: https://doi.org/10.1002/cca.2536

32. Menotti, A. & Puddu, P. E. How the Seven Countries Study contributed to the definition and development of the Mediterranean diet concept: A 50-year journey. *Nutrition, Metabolism and Cardiovascular Diseases*. 2015;25 (3):245–52. https://doi.org/10.1016/j.numecd.2014.12.001

33. Strisciuglio, C., Cenni, S., Serra, M. R., Dolce, P., Kolacek, S., Sila, S., et al. Diet and pediatric functional gastrointestinal disorders in Mediterranean countries. *Nutrients*. 2022;14(11):2335. https://doi.org/10.3390/nu14112335

34. Pieczyńska, K. & Rzymski, P. Health benefits of vegetarian and Mediterranean diets: narrative review. *Polish Journal of Food & Nutrition Sciences*. 2022;72(4):327–46. https://doi.org/10.31883/pjfns/156067

35. Trichopoulou, A. Mediterranean diet as intangible heritage of humanity: 10 years on. *Nutrition, Metabolism and Cardiovascular Diseases*. 2021;31 (7):1943–48. https://doi.org/10.1016/j.numecd.2021.04.011

36. Minelli, P. & Montinari, M. R. The Mediterranean diet and cardioprotection: historical overview and current research. *Journal of Multidisciplinary Healthcare*. 2019;12:805–15. https://doi.org/10.2147/JMDH.S219875

37. Burt, K. The whiteness of the Mediterranean diet: a historical, sociopolitical, and dietary analysis using critical race theory. *Journal of Critical Dietetics*. 2021;5(2):41–52. https://doi.org/10.32920/cd.v5i2.1329

38. Bach-Faig, A., Berry, E. M., Lairon, D., Reguant, J., Trichopoulou, A., Dernini, S., et al. Mediterranean diet pyramid today: science and cultural updates. *Public Health Nutrition*. 2011;14(12A):2274–84. https://doi.org/10.1017/s1368980011002515

39. Naureen, Z., Bonetti, G., Medori, M. C., Aquilanti, B., Velluti, V., Matera, G., et al. Foods of the Mediterranean diet: lacto-fermented food, the food pyramid and food combinations. *Journal of Preventive Medicine and Hygiene*. 2022;63(2 Suppl 3):E28–35. https://doi.org/10.15167/2421-4248/jpmh2022.63.2s3.2744

40. Michalak, L. & Trocki, K. Alcohol and Islam: an overview. *Contemporary drug problems*. 2006;33(4):523–62. https://doi.org/10.1177/009145090603300401

41. Kocturk, T. O. Food rules in the Koran. *Food & Nutrition Research*. 2002;1:137–39. https://doi.org/10.1080/11026480260363279

42. Hossein, S. M., Hassan, E. M., Babajafari, B. B., & Mazloomiand, S. M. Vegetarian and Western diets in Islam. *Europe – Revue Litteraire Mensuelle*. 2016:532–35.

43. Aboul-Enein, B. H. "The earth is your mosque": narrative perspectives of environmental health and education in the Holy Quran. *Journal of Environmental Studies and Sciences*. 2018;8:22–31. https://doi.org/10.1007/s13412-017-0444-7

44. Rahman, S. A. Religion and animal welfare: an Islamic perspective. *Animals*. 2017;7(2):11. https://doi.org/10.3390/ani7020011

45. Sahih Muslim. *Sahih Muslim 1955a*. In-book reference: Book 34, Hadith 84. Available from: https://sunnah.com/muslim:1955a

46. Tieman, M. Halal diets. *Islam and Civilisational Renewal*. 2016;274 (3399):1–5. https://doi.org/10.52282/icr.v7i1.295

47. Elgharbawy, A. & Azmi, N. A. Food as medicine: how eating Halal and Tayyib contributes to a balanced lifestyle. *Halalpshere*. 2022;2(1):86–97. https://doi.org/10.31436/hs.v2i1.39

48. Alzeer, J., Rieder, U., & Abou Hadeed, K. Rational and practical aspects of Halal and Tayyib in the context of food safety. *Trends in Food Science & Technology*. 2018;71:264–67. https://doi.org/10.1016/j.tifs.2017.10.020

Chapter

9

Recommended Eating and Dietary Practices in Islam

Nada Benajiba, MoezAllslam E. Faris, Lana Faiz Mahrous,
Hasnae Benkirane, Amina Bouziani, Yasmine Guennoun,
Basil H. Aboul-Enein

Introduction

Food choices and dietary habits play a crucial role in an individual's life and health. In many world religions, food is perceived as a source of pleasure, community, and rituals in addition to being a source of energy and nutrients for growth and development [1]. Thus, religion and spirituality through food choices and diet reflect a shared communal bond [2]. In Islam, food is viewed as a gift and blessing from Allah. The Holy Qur'an mentions "food," "eating," and "drink" 48 times, 107 times, and 39 times, respectively [3]. Consequently, the "act" of eating in Islam is perceived as a form of worship when food consumption is performed according to Islamic manners and teachings. In this regard, Islam recognizes the significance of food intake to nourish the body and mind. Hence, Islam provides dietary laws from the Holy Qur'an and Hadiths to guide Muslims on proper eating and drinking etiquettes [4].

Promoting Healthy, Balanced, and Diverse Food in Islam

Religion contributes significantly to shaping the population's diet, and the impact of religion on public health helps to identify and implement appropriate faith-based community intervention programs. Based on the well-established literature, healthy nutrition is related to the prevention of chronic diseases such as cardiovascular disease, diabetes, cancer, and obesity-related morbidities [5, 6, 7]. Islam supports the importance of nutrition and healthy eating [8]. Marzband et al. asserted that personal health can be reflected through observing Islamic teaching on food and eating practices [8, 9]. In Islam, there are 257 verses dealing with nutrition concepts in 70 out of 114 surahs in the Holy Qur'an [10]. For example, in Q Ar-Rahman 55:7–9, it says, "*And He enforced the balance. That you exceed not the bounds, but observe the balance strictly and fall not short thereof,*" which highlights the importance of avoiding or minimizing overindulgence and gluttony. Other verses that emphasize a healthy diet in the Holy Qur'an include Al-Baqarah 2:168, Al-An'am 6:141, and Ta-Ha 20:81 [11, 12, 13].

Previous studies have listed many different types of foods mentioned in the Holy Qur'an such as dates, grapes, pomegranates, figs, bananas, olives, olive oil, garlic, lentils, squashes, pumpkins, onions, milk, leafy vegetables, grain cereals, fish and seafood, poultry, and red meats, in addition to spices such as ginger, mustard, and basil [14, 15]. The emphasis encompasses different nutrition-related components such as diversity, moderation, and balance. Hence, the intake of nutrient-dense and *halal* (permitted) foodstuffs from an Islamic perspective is consistently promoted. In Q Al-Baqarah 2:168, Allah says, "*O mankind, eat from whatever is on earth [that is] lawful and good and do not follow the footsteps of Satan. Indeed, he is to you a clear enemy.*" Likewise, recommendations on fruits and vegetables, dairy, and protein consumption represent diet diversity which is aligned with international public health organizations such as the World Health Organization. Their recommendations include practical advice on maintaining a healthy diet based on consuming varied food groups [16]. Taken together, consuming food items from different food groups is referred to as dietary diversity which has long been considered as a key element of nutrient-dense dietary patterns [17]. Dietary diversity promotes adequate macro- and micronutrients; therefore, promoting food diversity is key to achieving appropriate nutrition-related health outcomes [18].

Eating in Moderation

In addition to moderation and diversity, principles of good nutrition include dietary balance. The term "balanced nutrition" means to meet the body's needs to ensure appropriate growth and maintenance by consuming a variety of foods that Allah has provided for all, including water, proteins, carbohydrates, fat, minerals, and vitamins [11, 12, 13]. One Qur'anic passage states, "*And He enforced the balance. That you exceed not the bounds, but observe the balance strictly, and fall not short thereof*" (Q Ar-Rahman 55:7–9). Dietary behavior in Islam also relies on the moderation concept. The Prophet Muhammad (PBUH) said the following:

> When filled with food, the belly becomes the worst container for the son of Adam. It is sufficient for a human being to have a few bites to keep himself fit (which means that it is sufficient to have only what one needs to maintain strength and well-being). If one must eat, then let him use one-third for food, one-third for drink, and one-third for breathing. [19]

According to evidence-based literature, moderation is the key to helping people maintain healthy and balanced lives [20, 21]. Studies have proven that excessive eating and an unhealthy diet can increase the risk of chronic diseases such as obesity, cardiovascular diseases, and diabetes [20, 21]. In addition, overeating has been discouraged in the Holy Qur'an: "*Eat and drink, but avoid excess*" (Q Ta-ha 20:81). Contemporary faith-based public health nutrition education programs could be designed by integrating the principles of good nutrition, balance, and moderation to complement other health-promoting programs to reduce the burden of nutrition-related chronic diseases in Muslim communities.

Eating Etiquettes in Islam

Islam, as a way of life, entails well-defined eating habits as a comprehensive guide for humankind. Islam as a doctrine provides a list of the food etiquettes involving social and emotional elements. Hence, many eating practices in Islam could be examined under the public health scope. For example, according to the Sunnah (teachings by the Prophet Muhammad [PBUH]), eating habits should be conceived with the perspective of helping to prevent ailments. In his saying, "When you drink (water or any liquid) do not breath in the vessel and when you urinate do not touch your private part with the right hand, and when you clean yourself after defecation, do not use your right hand" [22], the Prophet Muhammad (PBUH) considers personal hygiene and prevention of cross-contamination. Another saying by the Prophet Muhammad (PBUH) also insists on hand washing practices. It was narrated that "if he (the Prophet) wanted to eat or drink, he would wash his hands and then eat or drink" [23]. This is consistent with the international recommendations as reported by the CDC that hand washing is an effective method to reduce and prevent the spread of communicable diseases [24]. An international review study revealed that handwashing after contact with human excrement, such as urine and feces, is poorly practiced globally despite the positive public health impacts [25]. Of interest, then, is formulating such key messages based on Prophetic guidance into a religiously congruent reference frame for Muslim communities to integrate these practices into daily life.

Food Safety

Islam highlights human well-being as an important feature of Allah's worship. Islamic well-being encompasses physical, mental, and spiritual aspects. Ensuring such a principle as being clean is key for the believers in Islam, meaning the body, the clothes, the living place, and the food should all be clean. With this regard, food safety is treated under Islamic instructions because of its importance in ensuring that food is not contaminated with pathogenic agents in addition to knowing the behavioral principles of its consumption [26]. In the Holy Qur'an, there is clear direction for Muslims to pay attention to food, nutrition, and what they eat, ensuring that it is clean, *halal*, beneficial, and edible in all respects. One verse in the Qur'an states that people should keep away from every kind of destruction, including harm from unsafe food (Q Al-Baqarah 2:195). This supports the importance of food safety and sanitation. It could be understood as a prevention from and avoidance of any type of health risk caused by consuming contaminated and unsafe foods [27]. A systematic research study revealed that some selected community-based health education programs positively affect knowledge and attitude among the population with regard to food safety basics [28]. Biglari et al. recommended that health policymakers should consider the Islamic nutritional approach to achieve positive public health outcomes [3].

Conclusion

Teachings taken from the Holy Qur'an and Prophetic guidance could serve as a faith-based framework to develop culturally congruent public health intervention programs for Muslim communities. Relevant doctrines emphasizing healthy nutrition could serve as the base of culturally congruent initiatives at the individual, communal, or institutional levels to help populations achieve their maximum potential. The Islamic way of life could be perceived as a comprehensive basis, providing humankind with a set of complementary actions contributing to overall holistic well-being. Furthermore, a close evaluation of Qur'anic verses and the Prophet's guidance related to food and nutrition show that they are aligned with evidence-based guidelines and recommendations released by international authoritative organizations. Hence, public health care educators and practitioners could advocate effective interventions and health initiatives among practicing Muslim communities.

References

1. Robison, J. I., Wolfe, K., & Edwards, L. Holistic nutrition: nourishing the body, mind, and spirit. *Journal of Evidence-Based Integrative Medicine*. 2004;9 (1):11–20. https://doi.org/10.1177/1076167503252945

2. Shatenstein, B. & Ghadirian, P. Influences on diet, health behaviours and their outcome in select ethnocultural and

religious groups. *Nutrition.* 1998;14 (2):223–30. https://doi.org/10.1016/s0899-9007(97)00425-5

3. Biglari, H., Dargahi, A., Vaziri, Y., Ivanbagh, R., Hami, M., & Poursadeqiyan, M. Food safety and health from the perspective of Islam. *Journal of Pizhūhish dar dīn va salāmat.* 2020;6 (1):131–43. https://doi.org/10.22037/jrrh .v6i1.19142

4. Niri, S. A. Food health in the view of Islam. *Journal of Nutrition and Food Security.* 2021;6(3):262–71. https://doi .org/10.18502/jnfs.v6i3.6833

5. Sun, Y., You, W., Almeida, F., Estabrooks, P., & Davy, B. The effectiveness and cost of lifestyle interventions including nutrition education for diabetes prevention: a systematic review and meta-analysis. *Journal of the Academy of Nutrition and Dietetics.* 2017;117(3):404–21. https://doi .org/10.1016/j.jand.2016.11.016

6. Alexander, L., Christensen, S. M., Richardson, L., Ingersoll, A. B., Burridge, K., Golden, A., et al. Nutrition and physical activity: an obesity medicine association (OMA) clinical practice statement 2022. *Obesity Pillars.* 2022;1:100005. https://doi.org/10.1016/j .obpill.2021.100005

7. World Health Organization. Diet, nutrition, and the prevention of chronic diseases: report of a joint WHO/FAO expert consultation. [online]. 2002 [Accessed June 14, 2023]. Available from: www.who.int/publications/i/item/ 924120916X

8. Marzband, R. & Afzali, M. A. The role of nutrition in health with the approach of revelation. *Journal of Islamic and Iranian Traditional Medicine.* 2014;4(4):370–80.

9. Marzband, R., Moallemi, M., & Darabinia, M. Spiritual nutrition from the Islamic point of view. *Journal of Islamic Studies & Culture.* 2017;5(2):33–39.

10. Tarighat-Esfanjani, A. & Namazi, N. Nutritional concepts and frequency of foodstuffs mentioned in the Holy Quran. *Journal of Religion and Health.*

2016;55:812–19. https://doi.org/10.1007/ s10943-014-9855-x

11. Ghadimi, R., Kamrani, M., Zarghami, A., & Darzi, A. A. The role of nutrition in educational and spiritual development of human beings: Quranic perspective. *Journal of Babol University of Medical Sciences.* 2013;15(1):34–39.

12. Peyravi, D. & Moezzi, M. Healthy nutrition in Quran, the Muslim holy book. *International Proceedings of Chemical, Biological and Environmental Engineering (IPCBEE).* 2013;53:113–17.

13. Kocturk, T. O. Food rules in the Koran. *Food & Nutrition Research.* 2002;46 (3):137–39. http://dx.doi.org/10.1080/ 11026480260363279

14. Khafagi, I., Zakaria, A., Dewedar, A., & El-Zahdany, K. A voyage in the world of plants as mentioned in the Holy Quran. *International Journal of Botany.* 2006;2 (3):242–51. http://dx.doi.org/10.3923/ijb .2006.242.251

15. Shafaghat, A. Phytochemical investigation of Quranic fruits and plants. *Journal of Medicinal Plants.* 2010;9 (35):61–66.

16. World Health Organization. Healthy diet. [online]. 2020 [Accessed June 14, 2023]. Available from: https://www.who.int/ news-room/fact-sheets/detail/healthy-diet

17. Gonete, K. A., Tariku, A., Wami, S. D., & Akalu, T. Y. Dietary diversity practice and associated factors among adolescent girls in Dembia district, northwest Ethiopia, 2017. *Public Health Reviews.* 2020;41 (1):1–3. https://doi.org/10.1186/s40985- 020-00137-2

18. Verger, E. O., Le Port, A., Borderon, A., Bourbon, G., Moursi, M., Savy, M., et al. Dietary diversity indicators and their associations with dietary adequacy and health outcomes: a systematic scoping review. *Advances in Nutrition.* 2021;12 (5):1659–72. https://doi.org/10.1093/ advances/nmab009

19. Sunan Ibn Majah. *Sunan Ibn Majah 3349.* In-book reference: Book 29, Hadith 99. Available from: https://sunnah.com/ ibnmajah:3349

20. Martin, C., Zhang, Y., Tonelli, C., & Petroni, K. Plants, diet, and health. *Annual Review of Plant Biology*. 2013;29 (64):19–46. https://doi.org/10.1146/annurev-arplant-050312-120142

21. Krzyzanowska, J., Czubacka, A., & Oleszek, W. Dietary phytochemicals and human health. In: Giardi, M. T., Rea, G., & Berra, B., eds. *Bio-Farms for Nutraceuticals: Functional Food and Safety Control by Biosensors*. New York: Springer. 2010. 74–98.

22. Al Bukhari. *Sahih al-Bukhari 5630*. In-book reference: Book 74, Hadith 56. Available from: https://sunnah.com/bukhari:5630

23. Sunan an-Nasa'i. *Sunan an-Nasai 257*. In-book reference: Book 1, Hadith 258. Available from: https://sunnah.com/nasai:257

24. Allegranzi, B. & Pittet, D. Role of hand hygiene in healthcare-associated infection prevention. *Journal of Hospital Infection*. 2009;73(4):305–15. https://doi.org/10.1016/j.jhin.2009.04.019

25. Freeman, M. C., Stocks, M. E., Cumming, O., Jeandron, A., Higgins, J. P., Wolf, J., et al. Hygiene and health: systematic review of handwashing practices worldwide and update of health effects. *Tropical Medicine & International Health*. 2014;19(8):906–16. https://doi.org/10.1111/tmi.12339

26. Satin, M. *Food Alert!: The Ultimate Sourcebook for Food Safety*. New York: Facts On File, Inc. 2008.

27. Raheem, S. F. & Demirci, M. N. Assuring Tayyib from a food safety perspective in *halal* food sector: a conceptual framework. *MOJ Food Processing & Technology*. 2018;6 (2):170–79. https://doi.org/10.15406/mojfpt.2018.06.00161

28. Campbell, M. E., Gardner, C. E., Dwyer, J. J., Isaacs, S. M., Krueger, P. D., & Ying, J. Y. Effectiveness of public health interventions in food safety: a systematic review. *Canadian Journal of Public Health*. 1998;89:197–202. https://doi.org/10.1007/BF03404474

Chapter 10

Islamic Food Law and Dietary Restrictions

Elizabeth Dodge

Introduction

Cultural and religious teachings often guide food choice and food behavior and dictate religious-based dietary laws, thus having the potential to impact health [1–8]. There are over 1.8 billion Muslims worldwide, and Islam is considered the fastest-growing religion in the world [9]. Religious guidance on *halal* (permissible or acceptable) and *haram* (forbidden) foods is found in the Holy Qur'an and the Prophetic Hadith and informs practices regarding food selection, preparation, and the cleanliness of food [10]. Additional Qur'anic guidance is provided on food-related practices such as fasting, personal hygiene, sharing food, and breastfeeding [11–13].

Halal Foods, Breastfeeding, and Food Guidance

The Holy Qur'an provides numerous references to food, including 257 verses which address food and food practices [3]. Aboul-Enein relates 28 verses promoting healthful lifestyle practices including those around diet and nutrition and abstention from alcohol [13]. Some verses broadly approach food and food behavior, while others are very specific (such as Q Al-Baqarah 2:61; see also Table 10.1).

Breastfeeding is specifically promoted in the Holy Qur'an with guidance on the duration of breastfeeding, provisions for "wet nursing," and instruction on the father's role in supporting breastfeeding mothers (Q Al-Baqarah 2:61). The literature is supportive of breastfeeding as an Islamic human right, and multiple reviews have found essential public health benefits for both infants and mothers [14–18]. As it relates to breastfeeding, Qur'anic guidance can play a key role in maternal and infant health promotion [18–20] and could be used as a basis for initiatives to promote breastfeeding to Muslim populations [21–25].

Specific *halal* foods are also promoted in the Holy Qur'an, with 19 plants identified by name [3] including grains, cucumbers, alliums, lentils, grapes, olives, and dates [12–13, 26], and guidance is also provided on dairy, fish, and cattle [13]. Verses discussing specific *halal* foods, breastfeeding, and Qur'anic food guidance are included in Table 10.1.

Concepts of food diversity are proposed in the Holy Qur'an, which states, "*We can never endure one [kind of] food. So call upon your Lord to bring forth for us from the earth*" (Q Al-Baqarah 2:61). While some concern has been expressed about the potential for following religious dietary guidance leading to nutrient deficiencies, particularly in socio-economically disadvantaged populations, the Qur'anic guidance provided around food choice and *halal* foods aligns with the foundational tenets of a healthful diet [6, 11–13, 14].

Haram Foods and Food Guidance

Haram foods, or foods that are forbidden based on Qur'anic guidance, include carrion, blood, swine, predators, birds of prey, and animals that are not slaughtered in a *halal* manner [10]. Some verses addressing *haram* foods are included in Table 10.1. Alcohol is, in general, considered *haram* [11, 12, 26–27]. However, some consideration has been given to verses that may imply sparing use of alcohol is not *haram* in particular circumstances, such as under life-saving conditions as well as in the use of alcohol-based sanitizers, related to the tenet that "prevention is better than cure" [13, 28].

Qur'anic Guidance on *Halal* and *Haram* Foods: Illustrative Verses

Table 10.1 Selected Qur'anic verses on specific food items

Citation	Chapter: Verse
Halal *foods and food guidance*	
"It is lawful for you to hunt and eat seafood, as a provision for you and for travelers. But hunting on land is forbidden to you while on pilgrimage. Be mindful of Allah to Whom you all will be gathered."	(5:96)
"O humanity! Eat from what is lawful and good on the earth and do not follow Satan's footsteps. He is truly your sworn enemy."	(2:168)
"Eat from the good things We have provided for you, but do not transgress in them, or My wrath will befall you. And whoever My wrath befalls is certainly doomed."	(20:81)
"And within the land are neighboring plots and gardens of grapevines and crops and palm trees, [growing] several from a root or otherwise, watered with one water; but We make some of them exceed others in [quality of] fruit. Indeed in that are signs for a people who reason."	(13:4)
"And Verily! In the cattle, you have a worthy lesson. We give you to drink of that which is in their bellies, between the cud and blood: pure refreshing milk for those who drink it."	(16:66)
"And when you said, O Moses! We cannot endure one kind of food. Therefore, pray to your Lord to produce for us what the earth grows, its herbs, its cucumbers, its garlic, lentils, and onions."	(2:61)
"And caused to grow within it grains; and grapes and nutritious plants; and olives and dates; and gardens dense with many trees; and fruits and herbage."	(80:27–31)
Breastfeeding *and maternal care*	
"Mothers should breastfeed their children two complete years for whoever wishes to complete the nursing period."	(2:233)
"Upon the father is the mother's provision and their clothing according to what is acceptable."	(2:233)
Haram *foods and food guidance*	
"Prohibited to you are dead animals, blood, the flesh of swine, and that which has been dedicated to other than Allah, and [those animals] killed by	(5:3)

Table 10.1 (cont.)

Citation	Chapter: Verse
strangling or by a violent blow or by a head-long fall or by the goring of horns, and those from which a wild animal has eaten, except what you [are able to] slaughter [before its death]."	
"He has only forbidden to you dead animals, blood, the flesh of swine, and that which has been dedicated to other than Allah. But whoever is forced [by necessity], neither desiring [it] nor transgressing [its limit], there is no sin upon him. Indeed, Allah is Forgiving and Merciful."	(2:173)
"They ask you about wine and gambling. Say, 'In them is great sin and [yet, some] benefit for people. But their sin is greater than their benefit.' And they ask you what they should spend. Say, 'The excess [beyond needs].' Thus Allah makes clear to you the verses [of revelation] that you might give thought."	(2:219)

Halal Food Accessibility

Islamic food law upholds standards that promote the humane treatment of animals and describe how slaughtering animals for consumption should occur [29–32]. Practical implications of the industry may render current meat production techniques at odds with these standards, thereby creating a market for *halal* certification of meat products [33–36]. Issues and barriers related to *halal* certification have been identified, such as the need to implement *halal* practices through the whole food production and supply chain, appropriate transportation mechanisms to avoid cross-contamination with non-*halal* foods, the division among Islamic scholars on aligning Qur'anic guidance with modern slaughtering processes, and access to *halal* foods in some areas [31, 37–39]. While some literature has found that the use of *halal* certification may lead to an increase in business, serving as an incentive for businesses to offer *halal* foods [31, 36], literature also suggests *halal* certification can be cost-prohibitive for businesses, noting that the increase in cost may be passed along to consumers [34, 36, 40–42].

Accessibility to *halal* foods varies based on region and the factors listed above. Malaysia and Indonesia have been successful in promoting *halal* foods to Muslim tourists, and *halal* food is widely accessible there [32, 34–36, 38]. However, in non-Muslim majority countries and communities, *halal* foods can be less accessible and more difficult to find, which may result in food insecurity [43–47]. In areas where accessibility of *halal* foods is limited, there has been some adoption of technology to spread information to the wider Muslim community, connecting consumers with markets that offer *halal* options [48, 49, 50].

Islamic Food Law and Public Health Practice

Faith-based health promotion interventions have shown promising results related to lowering blood pressure, improving mental health, managing diabetes, and increasing physical activity [51–54]. Barriers to certain disparities such as food access and food insecurity can be mitigated through education and technology, and such initiatives could improve the health of minority Muslim and immigrant communities [43–50]. It has been found that by incorporating tenets of Islam and Qur'anic guidance in breastfeeding education and interventions, knowledge, support, and adoption of breastfeeding can be increased [18, 22–24]. Similarly, by incorporating Qur'anic guidance in health promotion initiatives, there could be important impacts on health-related behavior such as reducing adult and childhood obesity, reducing hesitancy of (and increasing adherence to) health screenings such as mammographies and colonoscopies, and reducing smoking [13, 55–57]. Public health practitioners should consider tailoring health-promotion interventions through a faith-based lens and include the voices of faith leaders and community members in the design and implementation of such initiatives to increase participation and intervention efficacy.

Conclusion

The Holy Qur'an provides food guidance to Muslims regarding what foods are considered *halal*, or permissible, versus those that are *haram*, or forbidden. Guidance on food selection and behaviors encourages a healthful approach to dietary components. The Qur'anic guidance around breastfeeding aligns with public health recommendations and could serve as a basis for interventions to increase breastfeeding rates and exclusivity in Muslim populations. Access to *halal* foods can be limited, especially in non-Muslim majority countries and communities, and has the potential to contribute to food insecurity. Particularly, immigrant Muslim populations can benefit from the use of social media or internet-based forums where they can share information that connects consumers to providers and markets.

References

1. Farouk, M. M., Regenstein, J. M., Pirie, M. R., Najm, R., Bekhit, A. E., & Knowles, S. O. Spiritual aspects of meat and nutritional security: perspectives and responsibilities of the Abrahamic faiths. *Food Research International.* 2015;76:882–95. https://doi.org/10.1016/j.foodres.2015.05.028

2. Bosire, E. N., Cele, L., Potelwa, X., Cho, A., & Mendenhall, E. God, church water and spirituality: perspectives on health and healing in Soweto, South Africa. *Global Public Health.* 2022;17(7):1172–85. https://doi.org/10.1080/17441692.2021.1919738

3. Khalid, S. M. N. & Sediqi, S. M. Improving nutritional and food security status in Muslim communities: integration of Quranic practices in development programs – a review. *International Journal of Nutrition Sciences.* 2018;3(2):65–72.

4. Ailin Qian. Delights in paradise: a comparative survey of heavenly food and drink in the Quran. In: Sebastian Günther & Todd Lawson, eds. *Roads to Paradise: Eschatology and Concepts of the Hereafter in Islam.* Vol. 1. Leiden: Brill. 2017. 251–70. https://doi.org/10.1163/9789004333154_012

5. Berry, E. M., Arnoni, Y., & Aviram, M. The Middle Eastern and biblical origins of the Mediterranean diet. *Public Health Nutrition.* 2011;14(12A):2288–95. https://doi.org/10.1017/s1368980011002539

6. Odukoya, O. O., Odediran, O., Rogers, C. R., Ogunsola, F., & Okuyemi, K. S. Barriers and facilitators of fruit and vegetable consumption among Nigerian adults in a faith-based setting: a pre-intervention qualitative inquiry. *Asian Pacific Journal of Cancer Prevention: APJCP.* 2022;23(5):1505–11. https://doi.org/10.31557/apjcp.2022.23.5.1505

7. Roudsari, A. H., Vedadhir, A., Amiri, P., Kalantari, N., Omidvar, N., Eini-Zinab, H., et al. Psycho-socio-cultural determinants of food choice: a qualitative study on adults in social and cultural context of Iran. *Iranian Journal of Psychiatry.* 2017;12(4):241.

8. Pakeeza, S. & Munir, M. Dietary laws of Islam and Judaism: a comparative study. *Al-Aẓvā*. 2016;31(45):1–4.

9. Lipka, M. Muslims and Islam: key findings in the US and around the world. [online]. Pew Research Center. 2017 [Accessed September 3, 2023]. Available from: https://pewrsr.ch/4dSVIE9

10. Farid, M. & Basri, H. The effects of *haram* food on human emotional and spiritual intelligence levels. *Indonesian Journal of Halal Research*. 2020;2(1):21–26. http://dx.doi.org/10.15575/ijhar.v2i1.7711

11. Kocturk, T. O. Food rules in the Koran. *Food & Nutrition Research*. 2002;1:137–39. https://doi.org/10.1080/11026480260363279

12. Hibban, M. F. Living Quran and Sunnah as the foundation of a holistic healthy lifestyle. *International Journal of Islamic and Complementary Medicine*. 2022;3 (2):49–56. https://doi.org/10.55116/IJICM.V3I2.40

13. Aboul-Enein, B. H. Health-promoting verses as mentioned in the Holy Quran. *Journal of Religion and Health*. 2016;55:821–29. https://doi.org/10.1007/s10943-014-9857-8

14. Chouraqui, J. P., Turck, D., Briend, A., Darmaun, D., Bocquet, A., Feillet, F., et al. Religious dietary rules and their potential nutritional and health consequences. *International Journal of Epidemiology*. 2021;50(1):12–26. https://doi.org/10.1093/ije/dyaa182

15. Dieterich, C. M., Felice, J. P., O'Sullivan, E., & Rasmussen, K. M. Breastfeeding and health outcomes for the mother-infant dyad. *Pediatric Clinics*. 2013;60(1):31–48. https://doi.org/10.1016/j.pcl.2012.09.010

16. Ip, S., Chung, M., Raman, G., Chew, P., Magula, N., DeVine, D., et al. Breastfeeding and maternal and infant health outcomes in developed countries. *Evidence Report/Technology Assessment*. 2007;(153):1–186.

17. Stuebe, A. The risks of not breastfeeding for mothers and infants. *Reviews in Obstetrics and Gynecology*. 2009;2 (4):222.

18. Bensaid, B. Breastfeeding as a fundamental Islamic human right. *Journal of Religion and Health*. 2021;60 (1):362–73. https://doi.org/10.1007/s10943-019-00835-5

19. Mehrpisheh, S., Memarian, A., Ameri, M., & Saberi, I. M. The importance of breastfeeding based on Islamic rules and Qur'an. *Hospital Practices and Research*. 2020;5(2):37–41. http://dx.doi.org/10.34172/hpr.2020.08

20. Firoozabadi, M. D. & Ali, M. S. Breastfeeding from Quran to medical science. *International Journal of Current Research and Academic Review*. 2015;3:134–37.

21. Bayyenat, S., Hashemi, S. A., Purbafrani, A., Saeidi, M., & Khodaee, G. H. The importance of breastfeeding in Holy Quran. *International Journal of Pediatrics*. 2014;2(4):339–47. https://doi.org/10.22038/ijp.2014.3396

22. Kamoun, C. & Spatz, D. Influence of Islamic traditions on breastfeeding beliefs and practices among African American Muslims in west Philadelphia: a mixed-methods study. *Journal of Human Lactation*. 2018;34(1):164–75. https://doi.org/10.1177/0890334417705856

23. Mohamad, E., Ahmad, A. L., Rahim, S. A., & Pawanteh, L. Understanding religion and social expectations in contemporary Muslim society when promoting breastfeeding. *Asian Social Science*. 2013;9(10):264. https://doi.org/10.5539/ass.v9n10p264

24. Kohan, S., Heidari, Z., & Keshvari, M. Facilitators for empowering women in breastfeeding: a qualitative study. *International Journal of Pediatrics*. 2016;4 (1):1287–96. http://dx.doi.org/10.22038/ijp.2016.6376

25. Saljughi, F., Savabi Esfahani, M., Kohan, S., & Ehsanpour, S. Promoting breastfeeding self-efficacy through role-playing in pregnant women. *International Journal of Pediatrics*. 2016;4(7):2061–68. https://doi.org/10.22038/ijp.2016.7000

26. Aboul-Enein, B. H. Reflections of the Holy Quran and the Mediterranean Diet:

a culturally congruent approach to obesity? *Mediterranean Journal of Nutrition and Metabolism.* 2015;8 (2):149–54. https://doi.org/10.3233/MNM-150041

27. Michalak, L. & Trocki, K. Alcohol and Islam: an overview. *Contemporary Drug Problems.* 2006;33(4):523–62. https://doi.org/10.1177/009145090603300401

28. Kashim, M. I. A. M., Majid, L. A., Adnan, A. H. M., Husni, A. B. M., Nasohah, Z., Samsudin, M. A., et al. Principles regarding the use of *haram* (forbidden) sources in food processing: a critical Islamic analysis. *Asian Social Science.* 2015;11(22):17–25. https://doi.org/10.5539/ass.v11n22p17

29. Rahman, S. A. Religion and animal welfare: an Islamic perspective. *Animals.* 2017;7(2):11. https://doi.org/10.3390/ani7020011

30. Abdullah, F. A., Borilova, G., & Steinhauserova, I. *Halal* criteria versus conventional slaughter technology. *Animals.* 2019;9(8):530. https://doi.org/10.3390/ani9080530

31. Farouk, M. M., Pufpaff, K. M., & Amir, M. Industrial *halal* meat production and animal welfare: a review. *Meat Science.* 2016;120:60–70. https://doi.org/10.1016/j.meatsci.2016.04.023

32. Benzertiha, A., Kierończyk, B. A., Rawski, M., Jozefiak, A., Mazurkiewicz, J., Jozefiak, D., et al. Cultural and practical aspects of *halal* slaughtering in food production. *Medycyna Weterynaryjna.* 2018;74(6):371–76. http://dx.doi.org/10.21521/mw.6023

33. Samori, Z., Ishak, A., & Kassan, N. H. Understanding the development of *halal* food standard: suggestion for future research. *International Journal of Social Science and Humanity.* 2014;4(6):482–86. http://dx.doi.org/10.7763/IJSSH.2014.V4.403

34. Nath, J., Henderson, J., Coveney, J., & Ward, P. Consumer faith: an exploration of trust in food and the impact of religious dietary norms and certification. *Food, Culture & Society.* 2013;16 (3):421–36. https://doi.org/10.2752/175174413X13673466711840

35. Henderson, J. C. *Halal* food, certification and *halal* tourism: insights from Malaysia and Singapore. *Tourism Management Perspectives.* 2016;19:160–64. https://doi.org/10.1016/j.tmp.2015.12.006

36. Fuseini, A., Wotton, S. B., Hadley, P. J., & Knowles, T. G. The compatibility of modern slaughter techniques with *halal* slaughter: a review of the aspects of "modern" slaughter methods that divide scholarly opinion within the Muslim community. *Animal Welfare.* 2017;26 (3):301–10. https://doi.org/10.7120/09627286.26.3.301

37. Zulfakar, M. H., Anuar, M. M., & Ab Talib, M. S. Conceptual framework on *halal* food supply chain integrity enhancement. *Procedia-Social and Behavioral Sciences.* 2014;121:58–67. https://doi.org/10.1016/j.sbspro.2014.01.1108

38. Jia, X. & Chaozhi, Z. Turning impediment into attraction: a supplier perspective on *halal* food in non-Islamic destinations. *Journal of Destination Marketing & Management.* 2021;19:100517. https://doi.org/10.1016/j.jdmm.2020.100517

39. Ab Talib, M. S., Abdul Hamid, A. B., & Ai Chin, T. Motivations and limitations in implementing *halal* food certification: a Pareto analysis. *British Food Journal.* 2015;117(11):2664–705. http://dx.doi.org/10.1108/BFJ-02-2015-0055

40. Ab Talib, M. S., Ai Chin, T., & Fischer, J. Linking *halal* food certification and business performance. *British Food Journal.* 2017;119(7):1606–18. http://dx.doi.org/10.1108/BFJ-01-2017-0019

41. Fuseini, A. *Halal* food certification in the UK and its impact on food businesses: a review in the context of the European Union. *CABI Reviews.* 2017;12(7):1–7. https://doi.org/10.1079/PAVSNNR201712007

42. Nuraini, S. Comparison *halal* food regulation and practices to support *halal* tourism in Asia: a review. *InIOP Conference Series: Earth and Environmental Science.* 2021;733:012044. http://dx.doi.org/10.1088/1755-1315/733/1/012044

43. Mansour, R., Liamputtong, P., & Arora, A. Food security among Libyan migrants living in Australia: a qualitative study. *Sustainability*. 2021;13(24):13853. https://doi.org/10.3390/su132413853

44. Lawlis, T., Islam, W., & Upton, P. Achieving the four dimensions of food security for resettled refugees in Australia: a systematic review. *Nutrition & Dietetics*. 2018;75(2):182–92. https://doi.org/10.1111/1747-0080.12402

45. Vatanparast, H., Koc, M., Farag, M., Garcea, J., Engler-Stringer, R., Qarmout, T., et al. Exploring food security among recently resettled Syrian refugees: results from a qualitative study in two Canadian cities. *International Journal of Migration, Health and Social Care*. 2020;16 (4):527–42. http://dx.doi.org/10.1108/IJMHSC-03-2019-0031

46. Goliaei, Z., Gonzalez, M., Diaz Rios, K., Pokhrel, M., & Burke, N. J. Post-resettlement food insecurity: Afghan refugees and challenges of the new environment. *International Journal of Environmental Research and Public Health*. 2023;20(10):5846. https://doi.org/10.3390/ijerph20105846

47. Moffat, T., Mohammed, C., & Newbold, K. B. Cultural dimensions of food insecurity among immigrants and refugees. *Human Organization*. 2017;76 (1):15–27. https://doi.org/10.17730/0018-7259.76.1.15

48. Kamarulzaman, Y., Veeck, A., Mumuni, A. G., Luqmani, M., & Quraeshi, Z. A. Religion, markets, and digital media: seeking *halal* food in the US. *Journal of Macromarketing*. 2016;36(4):400–411. https://doi.org/10.1177/0276146715622243

49. Mostafa, M. M. Global *halal* food discourse on social media: a text mining approach. *The Journal of International Communication*. 2020;26(2):211–37. https://doi.org/10.1080/13216597.2020.1795702

50. Mostafa, M. M. Information diffusion in *halal* food social media: a social network approach. *Journal of International Consumer Marketing*. 2021;33(4):471–91.

https://doi.org/10.1080/08961530.2020.1818158

51. Stella, S. Y., Wyatt, L. C., Patel, S., Choy, C., Dhar, R., Zanowiak, J. M., et al. A faith-based intervention to reduce blood pressure in underserved metropolitan New York immigrant communities. *Preventing Chronic Disease*. 2019;16:E106. https://doi.org/10.5888/pcd16.180618

52. Hays, K. & Aranda, M. P. Faith-based mental health interventions with African Americans: a review. *Research on Social Work Practice*. 2016;26(7):777–89. https://doi.org/10.1177/1049731515569356

53. Onyishi, C. N., Ilechukwu, L. C., Victor-Aigbodion, V., & Eseadi, C. Impact of spiritual beliefs and faith-based interventions on diabetes management. *World Journal of Diabetes*. 2021;12 (5):630. https://doi.org/10.4239/wjd.v12.i5.630

54. Bopp, M., Peterson, J. A., & Webb, B. L. A comprehensive review of faith-based physical activity interventions. *American Journal of Lifestyle Medicine*. 2012;6 (6):460–78. https://doi.org/10.1177/1559827612439285

55. Kotzur, M., Amiri, R., Gatting, L., Robb, K. A., Ling, J., Mooney, J. D., et al. Adapting participatory workshops to a virtual setting: co-design with Muslim women of a faith-based intervention to encourage cancer screening uptake. *International Journal of Qualitative Methods*. 2023;22:1–15. https://doi.org/10.1177/16094069231205194

56. Ismail, S., Abdul Rahman, H., Abidin, E. Z., Isha, A. S., Abu Bakar, S., Zulkifley, N. A., et al. The effect of faith-based smoking cessation intervention during Ramadan among Malay smokers. *Qatar Medical Journal*. 2017;2016(2):16. https://doi.org/10.5339/qmj.2016.16

57. Padela, A. I., Malik, S., Ally, S. A., Quinn, M., Hall, S., & Peek, M. Reducing Muslim mammography disparities: outcomes from a religiously tailored mosque-based intervention. *Health Education & Behavior*. 2018;45(6):1025–35. https://doi.org/10.1177/1090198118769371

Ramadan Intermittent Fasting: A Contemporary Health Perspective

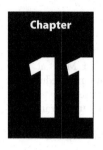

Meghit Boumediene Khaled, Mustapha Diaf, Maha H. Alhussain, MoezAlIslam E. Faris

Introduction

The holy month of Ramadan, the ninth month in the Islamic lunar calendar, is the sacred month during which all adult Muslims are mandated to refrain from eating, drinking, smoking, and doing sexual activities from dawn to sunset. Healthy adult Muslims are mandated to observe Ramadan fasting in response to the clear directions of the Holy Qur'an: "*O you who have believed, decreed upon you is fasting as it was decreed upon those before you that you may become righteous*" (Q Al-Baqarah 2:183). The Holy Qur'an also clearly states that Muslims have to fast if they are to remain righteous: "*But to fast is best for you, if you only knew*" (Q Al-Baqarah 2:184). In the same chapter of the Holy Qur'an, it states the following:

> *The month of Ramadhan [is that] in which was revealed the Qur'an, a guidance for the people and clear proofs of guidance and criterion. So whoever sights [the new moon of] the month, let him fast it; and whoever is ill or on a journey – then an equal number of other days. Allah intends for you ease and does not intend for you hardship and [wants] for you to complete the period and to glorify Allah for that [to] which He has guided you; and perhaps you will be grateful.*

> (Q Al-Baqarah 2:185)

Owing to the consistent fasting pattern for 29–30 consecutive days for 12–22 hours per day, different metabolic and physiological changes have been reported among healthy people and patients who opt to observe fasting during Ramadan [1]. Among the most prominently examined aspects are changes in body weight, circadian rhythm, cardiometabolic health, and the relationship with diabetes, which will be discussed further in this chapter.

Ramadan Intermittent Fasting and Body Weight Changes

The effect of Ramadan intermittent fasting (RIF) on body weight and composition is one of the most obvious and early-tested changes in RIF research, dating back to the 1980s [2]. To accurately estimate the effect size of body weight changes consequent to RIF, a recent systematic review and meta-analysis including 4,176 people aged 16–80 years reported a statistically significant yet small reduction in body weight (−1.022 kg). Fasting time duration (expressed in minutes per day) and solar season that crosses the lunar month were found to play significant roles in moderating the weight change at the end of Ramadan [3]. When it falls in the winter season, RIF is associated with a stable body weight or a slight increase in body weight by the end of Ramadan. Body composition, especially for total body fat mass and percentage, also showed variable changes at the end of the RIF month [4]. Fernando et al. examined the effect size of observing RIF on body fat composition [4]. Analysis of the 70 articles that included 2,947 participants showed a significant positive correlation between pre-fasting BMI and weight loss during Ramadan. In addition, a significant reduction in body fat percentage was observed between the pre- and post-Ramadan months in people with obesity. Further, the loss of fat-free mass was also significant between pre-Ramadan and post-Ramadan. However, this change in the body composition was transient, and the body weight and composition returned to their pre-fasting levels two to five weeks after Ramadan [4]. Recent research suggests gut microbiota plays a fundamental role in human health and disease, with obvious differences reported in the gut microbiota composition, diversity, and intestinal permeability between lean and obese people as well as in the same people upon body weight changes [5]. Within the large number of bacterial strains and types involved in the gut microbiota changes, increases in the relative abundance of *Akkermansia muciniphila*, which is known to be decreased in the gut of people with obesity [6], was evident through a recent systematic review and meta-analysis [5]. Such a change in *Akkermansia muciniphila* was reported upon the observance of RIF, as revealed by different reports [7, 8, 9].

Ramadan Intermittent Fasting, Circadian Rhythm, and Sleep

RIF is accompanied by profound changes in daily lifestyle routines, including feeding and sleeping patterns [10]. The timing of food and fluid intake during RIF suddenly shifts from daytime to darkness (the period between dawn and sunset). This practice partially delays the regular circadian pattern of feeding and thereby affects the circadian pattern of sleep [11]. A significant sudden delay in bedtime and waking time during Ramadan has been reported [12]. BaHammam et al. reported that bedtime was 1 hour and 18 minutes and 1 hour and 36 minutes later in the first and third weeks of Ramadan, respectively, compared with baseline (non-fasting) days [13]. Delayed bedtime during Ramadan was also observed among non-Muslims [13]. Further, RIF was found to affect sleep duration and daytime sleepiness. A systematic review and meta-analysis reported that there is an approximate one-hour reduction in sleep duration and approximately a one-point increase in the scale that measures daytime sleepiness during Ramadan compared with before Ramadan [10]. Attendant changes in day-night activity patterns that occur during Ramadan in some Muslim-majority countries, such as delays in starting school and work, stores and shopping malls remaining open until late at night, social gatherings with families and friends continuing until late at night, and voluntary prayers being conducted at night, were also proposed as potential causes of delay in circadian rhythms during Ramadan.

Although a delay in circadian rhythms is seen during Ramadan, a considerable body of evidence has demonstrated the beneficial effects of RIF on human health [4, 14, 15]. It should be noted that unique features of RIF, which includes the long, 30-day duration of the practice, might permit physiological adaptations to the new pattern. Thus, Ramadan eating and sleeping patterns differ from a nocturnal shift schedule and travel across multiple time zones, which have been linked to adverse health consequences due to circadian rhythm misalignment [16, 17]. Moreover, restricting food and hydration to a limited time of the day is predicted to result in lower energy intake [18]. During Ramadan, performers of fasting are ideally expected to consume two large meals – one in the early evening at sunset (*Iftar*) and the other in the early morning before dawn (*Suhour*) – and to have an adequate night's sleep. Restriction of mealtimes to the early evening and early morning hours, as well as getting a night of adequate sleep during Ramadan, had no effect on the circadian clock [19]. Furthermore, studies that controlled for the sleep/wake schedule, sleep duration, energy expenditure, and light exposure demonstrated no effect of fasting on circadian rhythms [12].

Cardiovascular and Cardiometabolic Health Implications

Between 1991 and 2012, several large retrospective, prospective, and case-control studies were undertaken in Muslim-majority countries such as Turkey, the Arab Gulf countries, and Albania to analyze the alteration of cardiovascular risk profiles during RIF in healthy subjects and in patients with stable heart disease, metabolic syndrome, dyslipidemia, type 2 diabetes (T2D), and systemic hypertension [20]. Major variations in metabolic and nutrient profiles during Ramadan may result from a combination of changes in lifestyle, sleep patterns, meal frequency, timing, and portioning, which are all combined into two meals per day. Additionally, these modifications may alter insulin resistance as well as several neurohormonal modifications associated with increased risk of developing cardiovascular disease (CVD) [21, 22]. A systematic review and meta-analysis on 4,431 adults aged 18–85 years suggested that RIF may improve cardiometabolic risk factors and have a short-term transient cardioprotective effect against CVD in healthy adults [23]. Further, inflammatory and oxidative stress markers that are known to predispose CVD, diabetes, and cancer are found to be ameliorated by the observance of RIF [24, 25], implying that observing RIF may entail a short-term transient protective effect against the development of CVD, diabetes, and cancer among healthy people. Examining the effect of observing RIF on high blood pressure, an important risk factor for heart failure, atrial fibrillation, and other cardiovascular complications, is important for elaborating the cardioprotective effect of RIF. In LORANS (London Ramadan Study), RIF revealed a positive effect on lowering blood pressure [26, 27]. Both systolic blood pressure (SBP) and diastolic blood pressure (DBP) were lowered in the latter two weeks of Ramadan or the first two weeks of *Shawaal* (the 10th month of the Islamic calendar) in the majority of the studies cited in the LORANS study, where SBP significantly decreased by 3.19 mm Hg, while DBP significantly decreased by 2.26 mm Hg [26]. This was also supported by two systematic reviews and meta-analyses that examined the effect of RIF on SBP and DBP among healthy people [14, 23].

Ramadan Intermittent Fasting and Diabetes

Fasting during Ramadan can be safe for patients with diabetes if they take some precautions and also may provide beneficial effects. RIF can be an opportunity to change one's lifestyle, decrease body weight, and change unhealthy behaviors. A recent systematic review and meta-analysis reported that RIF was significantly associated with favorable outcomes in patients with T2D such as causing an amelioration in glycemic control parameters [27]. As reported by the CREED study, a considerable proportion of the Muslim diabetic population was able to fast (63.6% completed the fast for the entire month) [9]. However, numerous studies reported that people with diabetes and health care professionals (HCPs) still face challenges during Ramadan. The sudden change in a regimented lifestyle includes a change in mealtimes and diet, sleep schedules, and physical activity habits [28]. In the EPIDIAR study, the major observed risks were hypoglycemia and hyperglycemia, which constituted challenges that diabetic patients face daily. Several studies showed that fasting may increase the occurrence of these complications. In type 1 diabetes and T2D patients, higher rates of severe hypoglycemia were recorded during Ramadan compared with before Ramadan [29]. Hence, categorization of patients and risk stratification as a pre-Ramadan evaluation become essential elements to consider by practitioners and diabetes organizations. The International Diabetes Federation (IDF) with the Diabetes and Ramadan Alliance (DAR) has recently published an updated version of guidelines evolving from the four tier categories in 2005 to the three-tier traffic light system (Category 1: very high risk; Category 2: high risk; Category 3: moderate/low risk), taking into consideration Ramadan-associated factors. Some factors related to Ramadan include length of fasting hours, season of fasting, weather, geographical location, social changes, and past experiences. Other factors are related to diabetes (type and duration of diabetes, complications, therapies, etc.) and individual dependents (i.e., age, sex, occupation, pregnancy, and motivation) [21, 28]. The DAR adopted a new approach and assigned a score to each risk element based on available evidence in the literature and clinical judgment. The approach corresponds to the basis of the religious regulations and principles of Islam. The following scores were adopted to every category (low risk: 0–3; moderate risk: 3.5–6; high risk: > 6), and therefore some recommendations on the ability/safety of fasting were provided. Despite all these recommendations, several diabetic individuals that are categorized as high risk still insist on fasting [21, 28]. A recent prospective study involving a relatively large population with T2D in the Middle East/North Africa region showed that about 90% fasted for ≥ 1 day, 86% fasted for ≥ 15 days, and 57% fasted for the full duration of Ramadan (30 days). Interestingly, significant improvements in body weight, HbA1C, and both fasting and postprandial blood glucose values were recorded in this study [30].

Conclusion

Safe fasting in Ramadan implies a need for a clear and defined knowledge of diabetes management and adaptations to self-monitoring of blood glucose schedules, medication intake, and culturally congruent education before engagement with RIF. Individuals with existing health conditions may be at greater risk of metabolic-related complications due to significant changes in food and fluid intake [31]. The challenges are to ensure that individuals with preexisting conditions who wish to fast can do so safely. Thus, public health educators and practitioners should help ensure patient safety with an evidence-based understanding of CVD, diabetes, and other health-related issues congruent with Ramadan that is needed along with an established set of guidelines to help inform culturally competent management strategies during Ramadan [28].

References

1. Faris, M. E., Assaad-Khalil, S. H., & Ali, T. What happens to the body? Physiology of fasting during Ramadan. In: Lessan, N., ed. *Diabetes and Ramadan Practical Guidelines 2021*. Brussels: International Diabetes Federation. 2021. 35–65.

2. Takruri, H. R. Effect of fasting in Ramadan on body weight. *Saudi Medical Journal*. 1989;10(6):491–94.

3. Jahrami, H. A., Alsibai, J., Clark, C. C., & Faris, M. E. A systematic review, meta-analysis, and meta-regression of the impact of diurnal intermittent fasting

during Ramadan on body weight in healthy subjects aged 16 years and above. *European Journal of Nutrition.* 2020;59 (6):2291–316. https://doi.org/10.1007/ s00394-020-02216-1

4. Fernando, H. A., Zibellini, J., Harris, R. A., Seimon, R. V., & Sainsbury, A. Effect of Ramadan fasting on weight and body composition in healthy non-athlete adults: a systematic review and meta-analysis. *Nutrients.* 2019;11(2):478. https://doi.org/10.3390/nu11020478

5. Koutoukidis, D. A., Jebb, S. A., Zimmerman, M., Otunla, A., Henry, J. A., Ferrey, A., et al. The association of weight loss with changes in the gut microbiota diversity, composition, and intestinal permeability: a systematic review and meta-analysis. *Gut Microbes.* 2022;14 (1):2020068. https://doi.org/10.1080/ 19490976.2021.2020068

6. Zhou, Q., Zhang, Y., Wang, X., Yang, R., Zhu, X., Zhang, Y., et al. Gut bacteria *Akkermansia* is associated with reduced risk of obesity: evidence from the American Gut Project. *Nutrition & Metabolism.* 2020;17(1):90. https://doi .org/10.1186/s12986-020-00516-1

7. Ali, I., Liu, K., Long, D., Faisal, S., Hilal, M. G., Ali, I., et al. Ramadan fasting leads to shifts in human gut microbiota structured by dietary composition. *Frontiers in Microbiology.* 2021;12:642999. https://doi.org/10.3389/ fmicb.2021.642999

8. Ozkul, C., Yalinay, M., & Karakan, T. Structural changes in gut microbiome after Ramadan fasting: a pilot study. *Beneficial Microbes.* 2020;11(3):227–33. https://doi.org/10.3920/bm2019.0039

9. Ozkul, C., Yalınay, M., & Karakan, T. Islamic fasting leads to an increased abundance of *Akkermansia muciniphila* and *Bacteroides fragilis* group: a preliminary study on intermittent fasting. *The Turkish Journal of Gastroenterology.* 2019;30(12):1030. https://doi.org/10 .5152/tjg.2019.19185

10. Faris, M. E., Jahrami, H. A., Alhayki, F. A., Alkhawaja, N. A., Ali, A. M., Aljeeb, S. H., et al. Effect of diurnal fasting on sleep

during Ramadan: a systematic review and meta-analysis. *Sleep and Breathing.* 2020;24(2):771–82. https://doi.org/10 .1007/s11325-019-01986-1

11. Bahammam, A. Effect of fasting during Ramadan on sleep architecture, daytime sleepiness and sleep pattern. *Sleep and Biological Rhythms.* 2004;2:135–43. https://doi.org/10.1111/j.1479-8425.2004 .00135.x

12. Qasrawi, S. O., Pandi-Perumal, S. R., & BaHammam, A. S. The effect of intermittent fasting during Ramadan on sleep, sleepiness, cognitive function, and circadian rhythm. *Sleep Breath.* 2017;21 (3):577–86. https://doi.org/10.1007/ s11325-017-1473-x

13. BaHammam, A. Assessment of sleep patterns, daytime sleepiness, and chronotype during Ramadan in fasting and nonfasting individuals. *Saudi Medical Journal.* 2005;26(4):616–22.

14. Faris, M. E., Jahrami, H. A., Alsibai, J., & Obaideen, A. A. Impact of Ramadan diurnal intermittent fasting on the metabolic syndrome components in healthy, non-athletic Muslim people aged over 15 years: a systematic review and meta-analysis. *British Journal of Nutrition.* 2020;123(1):1–22. https://doi .org/10.1017/s000711451900254x

15. Faris, M. E., Madkour, M. I., Obaideen, A. K., Dalah, E. Z., Hasan, H. A., Radwan, H., et al. Effect of Ramadan diurnal fasting on visceral adiposity and serum adipokines in overweight and obese individuals. *Diabetes Research and Clinical Practice.* 2019;153:166–75. https://doi.org/10.1016/j.diabres.2019.05 .023

16. Wang, F., Zhang, L., Zhang, Y., Zhang, B., He, Y., Xie, S., et al. Meta-analysis on night shift work and risk of metabolic syndrome. *Obesity Reviews.* 2014;15 (9):709–20. https://doi.org/10.1111/obr .12194

17. Nagata, C., Tamura, T., Wada, K., Konishi, K., Goto, Y., Nagao, Y., et al. Sleep duration, nightshift work, and the timing of meals and urinary levels of 8-isoprostane and 6-sulfatoxymelatonin in

Japanese women. *Chronobiology International*. 2017;34(9):1187–96. https://doi.org/10.1080/07420528.2017.1355313

18. Almeneessier, A. S. & BaHammam, A. S. How does diurnal intermittent fasting impact sleep, daytime sleepiness, and markers of the biological clock? Current insights. *Nature and Science of Sleep*. 2018;10:439–52.

19. BaHammam, A. S. & Almeneessier, A. S. Recent evidence on the impact of Ramadan diurnal intermittent fasting, mealtime, and circadian rhythm on cardiometabolic risk: a review. *Frontiers in Nutrition*. 2020;7:28. https://doi.org/10.3389/fnut.2020.00028

20. Salim, I., Al Suwaidi, J., Ghadban, W., Alkilani, H., & Salam, A. M. Impact of religious Ramadan fasting on cardiovascular disease: a systematic review of the literature. *Current Medical Research and Opinion*. 2013;29(4):343–54. https://doi.org/10.1185/03007995.2013.774270

21. International Diabetes Federation and DAR International Alliance. *Diabetes and Ramadan: Practical Guidelines 2021*. Brussels: International Diabetes Federation. 2021.

22. Almulhem, M., Susarla, R., Alabdulaali, L., Khunti, K., Karamat, M. A., Rasiah, T., et al. The effect of Ramadan fasting on cardiovascular events and risk factors in patients with type 2 diabetes: a systematic review. *Diabetes Research and Clinical Practice*. 2020;159:107918. https://doi.org/10.1016/j.diabres.2019.107918

23. Jahrami, H. A., Faris, M. E., Janahi, A. I., Janahi, M. I., Abdelrahim, D. N., Madkour, M. I., et al. Does four-week consecutive, dawn-to-sunset intermittent fasting during Ramadan affect cardiometabolic risk factors in healthy adults? A systematic review, meta-analysis, and meta-regression. *Nutrition, Metabolism and Cardiovascular Diseases*. 2021;31(8):2273–301. https://doi.org/10.1016/j.numecd.2021.05.002

24. Faris, M. E., Jahrami, H. A., Obaideen, A. A., & Madkour, M. I. Impact of diurnal intermittent fasting during Ramadan on inflammatory and oxidative stress markers in healthy people: systematic review and meta-analysis. *Journal of Nutrition & Intermediary Metabolism*. 2019;15:18–26. https://doi.org/10.1016/j.jnim.2018.11.005

25. Faris, M. E., Kacimi, S., Al-Kurd, R. A., Fararjeh, M. A., Bustanji, Y. K., Mohammad, M. K., et al. Intermittent fasting during Ramadan attenuates proinflammatory cytokines and immune cells in healthy subjects. *Nutrition Research*. 2012;32(12):947–55. https://doi.org/10.1016/j.nutres.2012.06.021

26. Al-Jafar, R., Zografou Themeli, M., Zaman, S., Akbar, S., Lhoste, V., Khamliche, A., et al. Effect of religious fasting in Ramadan on blood pressure: results from LORANS (London Ramadan Study) and a meta-analysis. *Journal of the American Heart Association*. 2021;10(20):e021560. https://doi.org/10.1161/jaha.120.021560

27. Elmajnoun, H. K., Faris, M. E., Abdelrahim, D. N., Haris, P. I., Abu-Median, A. B. Effects of Ramadan fasting on glycaemic control among patients with type 2 diabetes: systematic review and meta-analysis of observational studies. *Diabetes Therapy*. 2023;14(3):479–96. https://doi.org/10.1007/s13300-022-01363-4

28. Hassanein, M., Afandi, B., Ahmedani, M. Y., Alamoudi, R. M., Alawadi, F., Bajaj, H. S., et al. Diabetes and Ramadan: practical guidelines 2021. *Diabetes Research and Clinical Practice*. 2022;185:109185. https://doi.org/10.1016/j.diabres.2021.109185

29. Salti, I., Bénard, E., Detournay, B., Bianchi-Biscay, M., Le Brigand, C., Voinet, C., et al. A population-based study of diabetes and its characteristics during the fasting month of Ramadan in 13 countries: results of the epidemiology of diabetes and Ramadan 1422/2001 (EPIDIAR) study. *Diabetes Care*. 2004;27(10):2306–11. https://doi.org/10.2337/diacare.27.10.2306

30. Hassanein, M., Al Awadi, F. F., El Hadidy, K. E. S., Ali, S. S., Echtay, A., Djaballah, K., et al. The characteristics and pattern of care for the type 2 diabetes mellitus population in the MENA region during Ramadan: an international prospective study (DAR-MENA T2DM). *Diabetes Research and Clinical Practice*. 2019;151:275–84.

https://doi.org/10.1016/j.diabres.2019.02.020

31. Al-Arouj, M., Assaad-Khalil, S., Buse, J., Fahdil, I., Fahmy, M., Hafez, S., et al. Recommendations for management of diabetes during Ramadan: update 2010. *Diabetes Care*. 2010;33(8):1895. https://doi.org/10.2337/dc10-0896

Chapter 12

Promoting Oral Health: Influences of Hadith and Sunnah

Janine Owens, Sawsan Mustafa AbdallaSuliman

Introduction

This chapter discusses the importance of oral health promotion in the context of Islam. Globally, in increasingly multicultural societies, dental professionals need to possess insight into the cultural background of patients. Cultural diversity can produce different practices and views about oral health. These influencing factors include oral hygiene routines, diet, oral health beliefs, and access to care, all of which may affect oral health status. There is potential for a culturally informed focus and the creation of empowered communities by incorporating existing accepted guidance from the Prophetic Hadith and Sunnah into interventions. Muslim communities carry out their own traditional oral health practices, sometimes with alternatives to toothbrushes and toothpaste, as in the case of *Miswak*, a traditional dentifrice twig made from the *Salvadora persica* tree. The lack of acknowledgment by dental public health about diverse practices and guidance for Muslims makes it increasingly difficult to reorient oral health services. This acknowledgment is necessary in reducing inequalities and contributing towards a culturally competent pursuit of positive oral health.

Dentistry, the Mouth, and Oral Health Promotion

Separated from the body through the development of evidence-based research, the way the mouth is constructed and represented as an object for examination developed side by side with the new and emerging techniques of "normalization" [1, 2]. The process of normalization involves dentistry setting rules for the mouth such as correct techniques for brushing the teeth, the times when this should occur (morning and evening), and the space where this occurs (over a sink in a bathroom). Regular examination of the mouth occurs through dental checkups at regular intervals, measurements, and comparison through dental epidemiological surveys. Normalization (or the process of how the mouth becomes a normal everyday object) occurred through the categorization and placement of every mouth by comparing one to the next. This created ideals for the perfect mouth while also highlighting those that deviate away from perfection. So, for example, the name for the perfect aesthetics of the teeth and mouth is "the golden proportion," measured by the golden mean scale [3]. With knowledge of the mouth came the identification of disease and the need for individual oral health education, which was later followed by oral health promotion. Western dental public health frequently struggles with oral health promotion because its promoters lack cultural competence [4] and because Western communities focus on an upstream approach, ignoring the effects of oral health determinants and proposing that the individual alone can change the elements of their daily lifestyle [5]. However, for Muslims, oral hygiene practices reflect individual responsibility and are a part of practicing Islam [6]. Muslim refugees changing oral health practices and gravitating more towards adopting the cultural norms in their new country of domicile do not change their understanding of the need for oral hygiene, but, simultaneously, there is a feeling of cultural loss [7]. Another issue for Muslims moving to and settling in Western countries is diet. A change from a country of low- or middle-income status to one of high-income status can increase the availability of Western foods. Traditional diets are low in sugar, but frequently Western diets contain added sugars, which may result in worse oral and general health outcomes [7].

Oral diseases are a global public health problem and of particular concern in low- and middle-income countries (LMICs) because they link to rapidly changing socio-economic and commercial factors [8]. A focus on including Islamic beliefs and practices in oral health prevention and promotion for Muslim communities and refugees from LMICs settling in Western countries may help reduce oral health inequalities and result in more culturally competent care [9].

Impact of Poor Oral Health

Oral diseases affect people globally, creating a major health burden throughout their lifetime and causing discomfort, pain, disfigurement, or death [8]. They can also exert an effect on psychosocial outcomes [10] and self-image [11].

Major oral diseases are caries (tooth decay), periodontal conditions (gum disease) [12], head and neck cancer, and potentially malignant disorders [13]. Oral diseases share common risk factors with other major noncommunicable diseases (NCD) such as diabetes and cardiovascular disease, affecting general health and wellbeing [14]. Moreover, they link to social health determinants and, therefore, health inequalities [15]. The evidence that oral diseases link to common risk factors and the social determinants of health, alongside other NCDs, led to the inclusion of oral health in the World Health Organization (WHO) Health in All Policies (HiAP) [16, 17]. This moves the focus of oral health away from biomedical interventions and towards intersectoral partnerships [18] based on social justice, which considers the impact of the social determinants of health and acknowledges the influence of culture. Developed countries are attempting to tackle oral health inequalities; therefore, the implications of cultural diversity on national oral health promotion messages needs consideration. Generalized dental public health communications lack diversity and consideration for the oral health practices of different cultural groups [19]. This could inadvertently contribute to a widening of the gap in oral health inequalities.

Influence of Hadith and Sunnah on Oral Health

The Holy Qur'an is the main text of Islam. It is composed of 114 sections (surahs) containing unequal numbers and lengths of verses (*ayat*) [20]. Hadith is the reported words and deeds (Sunnah) of the Prophet (PBUH), which is considered the second source of knowledge and legislation in Islam [21]. It is significant to Muslims because it addresses ways of dealing with life, friends, family, government, and health, guiding all aspects of everyday life [21, 22]. The Sunnah covers all aspects of the lives of Muslims, but one aspect that does not receive much attention from Western public health is the focus of the Sunnah on personal hygiene, cleanliness, and health. The Sunnah has a holistic approach to health, viewing it in terms of the spiritual, physical, and cognitive alongside behaviors and practices.

Water has a particular significance in Islam. Before engaging in the five daily prayers, Muslims must carry out *wudu* (ablution). The Prophet (PBUH) guides Muslims to cleanse their mouths with water before praying and after each meal, particularly if they contain high levels of starches and fats. Leaving the tooth enamel exposed to high levels of sugars can cause dental decay [23], while leaving fatty substances in the mouth can cause bad breath (halitosis) [24].

Suwaid bin An Nu'man narrated the following:

> We went out with Allah's Messenger (PBUH) to Khaibar, and when we reached As-Sahba', the Prophet (PBUH) asked for food, and he was offered nothing but Sawiq (a meal made of wheat, rice, and barely). We ate, and then Allah's Messenger (PBUH) stood up for the prayer. He rinsed his mouth with water, and we too, rinsed our mouths.[25]

Further guidance is provided about contamination from saliva and about not drinking directly from the neck of water skins. Abu Sa'id Al-Khudri narrated, "I heard Allah's Messenger (PBUH) forbidding the drinking of water by bending the mouths of water skins, i.e., drinking from the mouths directly" [26]. The focus on hygiene and not contaminating the water or passing on potential oral pathogens to others appears implicit in this guidance.

The Prophet (PBUH) also encouraged Muslims to clean their mouths daily by using *Siwāk*. *Siwāk* or *Miswak* comes from the *Salvadora Persica* tree (*Arāk* in Arabic) and refers to a small wooden stick which, when soaked in water and then chewed, creates bristle-like strands that help to remove food debris from the teeth, freshen the mouth, protect tooth enamel, and promote gingival wound healing with its antibacterial and anti-cariogenic properties [27]. Within the Hadith are numerous mentions of *Miswak* [28].

Table 12.1 illustrates the 51 Hadiths mentioning *Miswak*, taken from the two books (Sahih al-Bukhari and Sahih Muslim) of the most authentic references of the Hadith of the Prophet (PBUH). Authenticity refers to the proposed criteria that must occur for each narrative (*matn*) in the chain of Hadith narrations (*isnad*) and which form a foundation for their inclusion [29].

Table 12.1 Hadith mentioning *Miswak*

No.	Name of Hadith about *Miswak*	Book of Hadith	Total number of Hadith
1.	Sahih al-Bukhari	Book of Ablution, Book of Jumaat, Book of Tahajjud, Book of Prayer, Book of Five Compulsory (Fardhu al-Khams), Book of Fasting, Friday Prayer, Book of Wishes, Military Expeditions led by the Prophet (PBUH), Prophetic Commentary on the Holy Qur'an, Book of Dealing with Apostates, One-fifth of Booty to the Cause of Allah (Khumus)	30
2.	Sahih Muslim	Book of Hygiene (Taharah), Chapter of Siwak, Book of Prayer, Book of Juma'at, Book of Hajj, Book of Ru'yah, Book on Government	21

The Hadiths contain guidance on how and when to use *Miswak* and its benefits and importance. One Hadith stated, "I came to the Prophet (PBUH) and I saw him carrying a Siwak in his hand and cleaning his teeth, saying, 'u' u" as if he was retching while the Siwak was in his mouth" [30]. Abu Musa Al-Ash'ari also reported, "I came to the Prophet (PBUH) once and noticed the tip of *Miswak* (tooth-stick) on his tongue" [31]. These two excerpts from the Hadith offer guidance on how to use *Miswak* for cleaning the teeth and tongue. Research suggests that *Miswak* is effective for removing dental plaque and is comparable to a toothbrush [32]. It further suggests that although Muslims are aware of Prophetic traditions in the Hadith about *Miswak*, they are unsure as to the reasons why [29]. The recommended guidance on *Miswak* use include the following: before each of the five prayer calls, while performing *wudu*, before the recitation of the Qur'an, upon awakening, when entering a mosque or house, and when interacting with others [33]. *Fluoridated Miswak* use would remove acid-producing bacterial microorganisms and leaves a protective layer of fluoride on the teeth [34, 35].

However, the Prophet (PBUH) displayed awareness about not enforcing the use of *Miswak* before every prayer call by considering that Muslims may be unable to perform the practice regularly. Allah's Messenger (PBUH) said, "Were I not afraid that it would be hard on my followers, I would order them to use the Siwak (as obligatory, for cleaning the mouth and the teeth)" [36].

According to Abu Huraira, the Prophet (PBUH) said, "(Allah said), 'Every good deed of Adam's son is for him except fasting; it is for Me. and I shall reward (the fasting person) for it.' Verily, the smell of the mouth of a fasting person is better to Allah than the smell of musk" [37]. Using *Miswak* stimulates the production of saliva, which is a buffering agent and protects the teeth against bacterial and fungal organisms [38]. For example, saliva in conjunction with the antioxidants within *Miswak* acts as a protective agent against fungal infections such as *Candida albicans* and enterococcal infections [39]. Its mild analgesic effect is useful in reducing oral pain, which often occurs when periodontal (gum) disease is present – particularly for people with diabetes, who can also be at risk for xerostomia (dry mouth). Some studies suggest a significantly greater reduction of gingivitis (inflamed and bleeding gums) when using *Miswak* mouthwash compared to chlorhexidine [24]. Left unchecked, periodontal disease may lead to loosened teeth or tooth loss, which then has implications for nutrition because of the reduction in ability to masticate, thus rendering some foods impossible to eat. This dietary change then exerts an effect on general health.

Oral health is a precursor to general health. The Holy Qur'an tasks Muslims to take care of their bodies, viewing the mouth holistically as part of the body, not separate, and therefore in need of maintenance by whatever means necessary, including by seeking treatment. *Miswak* in any of its forms, whether as a stick or as any of the modern forms of toothbrush and toothpaste, is part of prophetic guidance for cleaning the teeth and mouth and can therefore be utilized as a holistic tool for maintaining positive oral and general health. This makes *Miswak* a culturally inclusive, natural, ecologically friendly, and inexpensive way of maintaining oral hygiene [40].

One barrier to the use of *Miswak* is the rise of Westernized practices such as the use of a toothbrush and toothpaste with some cultural groups who view possession of a toothbrush as denoting status and wealth [41]. While this symbolism is to some extent positive, it may simultaneously exert negative effects because of the lack of oral health literacy and understanding of oral hygiene. For example, the biggest preventive achievement for oral health is fluoride in the form of fluoridated toothpaste, which is a protective factor against dental caries. Fluoridated toothpaste is regulated and affordable in high-income countries, but in LMICs it is unregulated, of poor quality (often lacking in fluoride), and unaffordable [42]. This makes it challenging to improve the oral health outcomes of people living in socioeconomically deprived areas. Another barrier is the lack of acknowledgment or understanding of the evidence-based literature from dental public health practitioners for the oral health practices of Muslims, *Miswak* use, and Islamic principles involving oral hygiene [19].

Conclusion

When developing culturally congruent messages promoting oral hygiene, dental public health practitioners need to acknowledge that alternative oral hygiene aids and practices play a significant role for Muslims worldwide. With the rise in refugees and migrant groups globally who often experience marginalization and disadvantage, the discipline of dental public health needs to understand, respect, and incorporate different cultural practices for oral health care alongside policies to reduce the significant oral health inequalities experienced in diverse cultures. Incorporating guidance from the Holy Qur'an, Hadith, and Sunnah may assist with this challenge.

References

1. Nettleton, S. Protecting a vulnerable margin: towards an analysis of how the mouth came to be separated from the body. *Sociology of Health and Illness.* 1988;10:156–69. https://doi.org/10.1111/1467-9566.ep11339934

2. Nettleton, S. Power and pain: the location of pain and fear in dentistry and the creation of a dental subject. *Social Science & Medicine.* 1989;29:1183–90. https://doi.org/10.1016/0277-9536(89)90361-4

3. Londono, J., Ghasemi, S., Lawand, G., & Dashti, M. Evaluation of the golden proportion in the natural dentition: a systematic review and meta-analysis. *Journal of Prosthetic Dentistry.* 2021;129 (5):696–702. https://doi.org/10.1016/j.prosdent.2021.07.020

4. Laverack, G. Is health promotion culturally competent to work with migrants? *Global Health Promotion.* 2018;25(2):3–5. https://doi.org/10.1177/1757975918777688

5. Daly, B., Watt, R. G., Batchelor, P., & Treasure, E. Definitions of health. In: Daly, B., Batchelor, P., Treasure, E., & Watt, R G., eds. *Essential Dental Public Health.* 2nd Ed. Oxford: Oxford University Press. 2013. 23–36.

6. Beveridge, S. Oral health beliefs, traditions and practices in the Somali culture. *Oral Health.* 2001;2(1):1–5.

7. Adams, J. H., Young, S., Laird, L. D., Geltman, P. L., Cochran, J. J., Hassan, A., et al. The cultural basis for oral health practices among Somali refugees, pre-and post-resettlement in Massachusetts. *Journal of Health Care for the Poor and Underserved.* 2013;24(4):1474–85. https://doi.org/10.1353/hpu.2013.0154

8. Peres, M. A., Macpherson, L. M. D., Weyant, R. J., Daly, B., Venturelli, R., Mathur, M. R., et al. Oral diseases: a global public health challenge. *The Lancet.* 2019;394(10194):249–60. https://doi.org/10.1016/S0140-6736(19)31146-8

9. Sirois, M., Darby, M., & Tolle, S. Understanding Muslim patients: cross-cultural dental hygiene care. *International Journal of Dental Hygiene.* 2013;11:105–14. https://doi.org/10.1111/j.1601-5037.2012.00559.x

10. Locker, D., Clarke, M., & Payne, B. Self-perceived oral health status, psychological well-being, and life satisfaction in an

older adult population. *Journal of Dental Research.* 2000;79(4):970–75. https://doi.org/10.1177/00220345000790041301

11. Malekpour, P., Devine, A., Dare, J., & Costello, L. Investigating the perspectives of older adults in residential aged care on oral health-related quality of life. *Gerodontology.* 2022;40(2):220–30. https://doi.org/10.1111/ger.12636

12. Marcenes, W., Kassebaum, N. J., Bernabé, E., Flaxman, A., Naghavi, M., Lopez, A., et al. Global burden of oral conditions in 1990–2010: a systematic analysis. *Journal of Dental Research.* 2013;92(7):592–97. https://doi.org/10.1177/0022034513490168

13. Ren, Z. H., Hu, C. Y., He, H. R., Li, Y. J., & Lyu, J. Global and regional burdens of oral cancer from 1990 to 2017: results from the global burden of disease study. *Cancer Communications.* 2020;40(2–3):81–92. https://doi.org/10.1002/cac2.12009

14. Jin, L. J., Lamster, I. B., Greenspan, J. S., Pitts, N. B., Scully, C., & Warnakulasuriya, S. Global burden of oral diseases: emerging concepts, management and interplay with systemic health. *Oral Diseases.* 2016;22(7):609–19. https://doi.org/10.1111/odi.12428

15. Kwan, S. & Petersen, P. E. Oral health: equity and social determinants. In: Blas, E. & Sivasankara Kurup, A., eds. *Equity, Social Determinants and Public Health Programmes.* Geneva: World Health Organization. 2010. 159–76.

16. World Health Organization. *Adelaide Statement on Health in All Policies.* Adelaide: World Health Organization, Government of South Australia. 2010.

17. World Health Organization. *Adelaide Statement II on Health in All Policies.* Adelaide: World Health Organization, Government of South Australia. 2019.

18. Meier, B. M., Brodish, P. H., & Koivusalo, M. Human rights provide justification for the Health in All Policies. [online]. Health and Human Rights. 10 June 2013 [Accessed April 4, 2023]. Available from: www.hhrjournal.org/2013/06/human-rights-provide-justification-for-the-health-in-all-policies-approach/

19. Riggs, E., van Gemert, C., Gussy, M., Waters, E., & Kilpatrick, N. Reflections on cultural diversity in oral health promotion and prevention. *Global Health Promotion.* 2012;19(1):60–63. https://doi.org/10.1177/1757975911429872

20. Al-Laithy, A. *What Everyone Should Know About the Qur'an.* Antwerp, BE: Garant Uitgevers NV. 2005.

21. Elkadi, A. Health and healing in the Qur'an. *American Journal of Islam and Society.* 1985;2(2):291–96. https://doi.org/10.35632/ajis.v2i2.2771

22. Alfarisi, H., Osmani, N. M., & Zubi, Z. The status of Sunnah in Islam. *International Journal of Academic Research in Business and Social Sciences.* 2023;13(2):663–69. http://dx.doi.org/10.6007/IJARBSS/v13-i2/16292

23. Moynihan, P. Diet and dental caries. In: Murray, J., Nunn, J., & Steele, J. G., eds. *The Prevention of Oral Disease.* Oxford: Oxford University Press. 2003. 7–34

24. Van Der Weijden, F. & Slot, D. E. Oral hygiene in the prevention of periodontal diseases: the evidence. *Periodontology 2000.* 2011;55(1):104–23. https://doi.org/10.1111/j.1600-0757.2009.00337.x

25. Sahih al-Bukhari. *Sahih al-Bukhari 5454.* In-book reference: Book 70, Hadith 83. Available from: https://sunnah.com/bukhari:5454

26. Sahih al-Bukhari. *Sahih al-Bukhari 5626.* In-book reference: Book 74, Hadith 52. Available from: https://sunnah.com/bukhari:5626

27. Nordin, A., Rahim, A. Z., Abdul Razzak, M. M., & Bakri, M. M. The practice of using chewing stick (*Salvadora persica*) in maintaining oral health: knowledge, perception and attitude of Malaysian Muslims adult. *World Applied Sciences Journal.* 2014;30(30):351–59.

28. Owens, J. & Sami, W. The role of the Qur'an and Sunnah in oral health. *Journal of Religion and Health.* 2016;55:1954–67. https://doi.org/10.1007/s10943-015-0095-5

29. Musa, A. Y. *Hadith as Scripture: Discussions on The Authority Of Prophetic*

Traditions in Islam. New York: Palgrave. 2008.

30. Sahih al-Bukhari. *Sahih al-Bukhari 244.* In-book reference: Book 4, Hadith 110. Available from: https://sunnah.com/ bukhari:244

31. Riyad as-Salihin. *Riyad as-Salihin 1201.* In-book reference: Book 8, Hadith 211. Available from: https://sunnah.com/ riyadussalihin:1201

32. Nordin, A., Bin Saim, A., Ramli, R., Abdul Hamid, A., Mohd Nasri, N. W., & Bt Hj Idrus, R. Miswak and oral health: an evidence-based review. *Saudi Journal of Biological Sciences.* 2020;27(7):1801–10. https://doi.org/10.1016/j.sjbs.2020.05.020

33. Rispler-Chaim, V. The Siwāk: a medieval Islamic contribution to dental care. *Journal of the Royal Asiatic Society.* 1992;2 (1):13–20. https://doi.org/10.1017/ S1356186300001772

34. Baeshen H, Salahuddin S, Dam R, Zawawi KH, Birkhed D. Comparison of fluoridated Miswāk and toothbrushing with fluoridated toothpaste on plaque removal and fluoride release. *J. Contemp. Dent. Pract.* 2017, 18(4): 300–306. https:// 10.5005/jp-journals-10024-2035

35. Malik, A. S., Shaukat, M. S., Qureshi, A. A., & Abdur, R. Comparative effectiveness of chewing stick and toothbrush: a randomized clinical trial. *North American Journal of Medical Science.* 2014;6:333–37. https://doi.org/10 .4103/1947-2714.136916

36. Sahih al-Bukhari. *Sahih al-Bukhari 7240.* In-book reference: Book 94, Hadith 15.

Available from: https://sunnah.com/ bukhari:7240

37. Sahih al-Bukhari. *Sahih al-Bukhari 5927.* In-book reference: Book 77, Hadith 142. Available from: https://sunnah.com/ bukhari:5927

38. Nassar, M., Hiraishi, N., Islam, M. S., Otsuki, M., & Tagami, J. Age-related changes in salivary biomarkers. *Journal of Dental Sciences.* 2014;9 (1):85–90. https://doi.org/10.1016/j.jds .2013.11.002

39. Balto, H., Al-Howiriny, T., Al-Somily, A., Siddiqui, Y. A., Al-Sowygh, Z., Halawany, H., et al. Screening for the antimicrobial activity of *Salvadora persica* extracts against *Enterococcus faecalis* and *Candida albicans. International Journal of Phytomedicine.* 2013;5(4):486–92.

40. Mohamed, S. A. & Khan, J. A. Antioxidant capacity of chewing stick *Miswak Salvadora persica. BMC Complementary and Alternative Medicine.* 2013;13:40. https://doi.org/10.1186/1472- 6882-13-40

41. Owens, J. & Saeed, S. M. Exploring the oral health experiences of a rural population in Sudan. *International Dental Journal.* 2008;58(5):258–64. https://doi .org/10.1111/j.1875-595X.2008.tb00197.x

42. Gkekas, A., Varenne, B., Stauf, N., Benzian, H., & Listl, S. Affordability of essential medicines: the case of fluoride toothpaste in 78 countries. *PLoS ONE.* 2022;17(10):e0275111. https://doi.org/10.1371/journal.pone .0275111

Chapter 3

Coping and Mental Health: Islamic Practices and Beliefs

G. Hussein Rassool, Janine Owens

Introduction

Muslims believe the Holy Qur'an is the divine word of Allah. They believe reciting and listening to these words brings tranquility and peace to their minds and hearts. The Qur'an maintains a balance between different aspects of human life, and Islamic medicine uses the Holy Qur'an to promote health and treat people with psychological disorders [1, 2]. Traditionally, the global Islamic community (*Ummah*) plays an important role in supporting Muslims in many different ways, such as firstly providing emotional support and secondly forming a crucial link between government authorities and Muslims [3].

Despite the growth of Islam globally, within their educational and clinical preparations Western medical practitioners appear to lack insight into Islamic culture, values, and teachings [4]. Furthermore, research suggests some Muslims are unwilling to seek help for mental health difficulties in Western countries because of mental health professionals' belief differences and their lack of understanding of the importance of Islamic values in treatment planning [5, 6, 7]. Other research details the influence of Western paradigms and discourses on health care systems, nursing care, and management in both non-Islamic and Islamic countries, which excludes the needs and experiences of Muslims [8, 9]. This lack of cultural competence could be a barrier for Muslims who may avoid seeking mental health assistance because it conflicts with their religious and spiritual beliefs.

Religious and Spiritual Coping

Religious and spiritual coping is defined as "process that people engage in to attain significance in stressful circumstances" [10]. Religious coping strategies often stem directly from religious belief systems and enable individuals to construct and interpret meanings in different situations. Religious coping can be positive or negative. Positive religious coping occurs when people believe that their God is guiding them and displays positive outcomes because whatever happens is by the will of their God [11]. This type of coping also enables spiritual growth. In contrast, negative religious coping occurs when people feel abandoned by God and increases negative outcomes including anxiety, elevated stress, depression, and somatization [12]. Muslims structure their everyday lives and religious practices around Allah, believing that whatever happens, it is His will. Placing their faith in Him strengthens their belief and enhances their relationship with Allah. Allah says in the Holy Qur'an, "*And for those who fear Allah, He always prepares a way out, and He provides for him from sources he never could imagine. And if anyone puts his trust in Allah, sufficient is Allah for him. For Allah will surely accomplish His purpose: verily, for all things has Allah appointed a due proportion"* (Q Aṭ-Ṭalaq 65:3).

Biopsychosocial Model of Care and Islam

Within Western psychiatry and psychology, a shift away from a reductionist biomedical model (where health and illness are viewed in terms of medically defined pathology) to a biopsychosocial (BPS) model of care gained greater adherence from 1977 onward, beginning with seminal work by Engel who argued against a Cartesian divide [13]. The BPS model of care is a more holistic patient approach that considers the interaction of psychosocial and biological factors as essential for diagnosis and care [14]. However, the BPS model of care still splits religion and spirituality into two different constructs, whereas Islam views religion and spirituality as mutually intertwined where one cannot exist without the other [15]. Research argues that Islam enables Muslims to cope with everyday life, especially when challenges occur, assisting in reducing levels of anxiety and reactive depression [16, 17]. This indicates the use of positive religious coping, which is positively associated with desirable mental health and well-being indicators in contrast with negative religious coping [14].

Positive Religious Coping and Islam

Muslims turn to Allah in their time of distress and grief. The life story of the Prophet Muhammad (PBUH) and the multiple losses of his loved ones are all teachings for dealing with grief, as are Hadiths and surah from the Qur'an. Allah says in the Qur'an, *"Allah leaves astray whom He wills and guides to Himself whoever turns back [to Him] – those who have believed and whose heart are assured by the remembrance of Allah. Unquestionably, by the remembrance of Allah, hearts are assured"* (Q Ar-Ra'd 13:27–28). Muslims believe that life, death, joy, grief, and happiness emanate from Allah, and any deprivation or negative experience is a test from Allah to identify the strength of their faith. Allah also says in the Qur'an, *"Be sure we shall test you with something of fear and hunger, some loss in goods, lives, and the fruits of your toil, but give glad tiding to those who patiently persevere. Who say, when afflicted with calamity: To Allah we belong, and to Him is our return"* (Q Al-Baqarah 2:155–56). This type of belief develops greater acceptance in the face of adversity, enabling positive coping to occur. For example, when experiencing the death of a loved one, Muslims are encouraged to talk about and remember them and their good deeds throughout their lives. An example of this in the Holy Qur'an is the Prophet Muhammad (PBUH) discussing his beloved wife, Khadijah, years after her death and the jealousy of his wife Aisha [18]. Al-Bukhari entitled a chapter in his Sahih "The marriage of the Prophet (PBUH) to Khadijah (may Allah be pleased with her), and her virtues," in which he narrated a Hadith from Aisha who said, "I never felt jealous of any of the wives of the Prophet (PBUH) as I did of Khadijah, although she died before he married me, because of what I heard him say about her" [19].

Islamic Coping Mechanisms

The purposes of the Islamic coping mechanisms encompass a range of practices aimed at finding solace, seeking guidance, and strengthening one's faith during challenging times.

Some of the Islamic coping mechanisms practiced by Muslims include *dhikr* (mentioning and reciting the name of Allah), *salah* (prayer), Qur'anic recitation, patience and acceptance, *istighfar* (seeking forgiveness), and *sadaqah* (charitable acts).

Dhikr refers to the remembrance of Allah through repetitive recitation of His 99 names and supreme attributes, specific phrases, or verses of the Holy Qur'an. It is a form of devotion to Allah and is divided into three forms: "the first is *dhikr* with heart, the second is *dhikr* with oral (speech), and the third is *dhikr* with deeds" [20]. Ibn Al-Qayyim refers to *dhikr* as "any and every particular moment when you are thinking, saying or doing things which Allah likes" [21].

It is a form of contemplation where Muslims engage in the constant remembrance of Allah; the aims are to purify their hearts, find inner peace, strengthen their faith, protect them from evil, and enable them to cope with trials and tribulations [22, 23]. The Prophet Muhammad (PBUH) said in *Hadith Qudsi*,

> Allah says: "I am just as My slave thinks I am, (i.e., I am able to do for him what he thinks I can do for him) and I am with him if he remembers Me. If he remembers Me in himself, I too, remember him in Myself; and if he remembers Me in a group of people, I remember him in a group that is better than they; and if he comes one span nearer to Me, I go one cubit nearer to him; and if he comes one cubit nearer to Me, I go a distance of two outstretched arms nearer to him; and if he comes to Me walking, I go to him running." [24]

Some of the *dhikr* include *Alhamdullilah* (All Praise is for Allah), *SubhanAllah* or *SubhanAllah wa Bihamdihi* (Glory to Allah and Praise Him), *SubhanAllah wal hamdillilah* (Glory to Allah and praise be to Allah), and *Allah Hu Akbar* (Allah is great). According to Imam an-Nawawi, there are many virtues of *dhikr* and encouragement to remember Allah in the following Qur'anic verses: Q Al-Ankabut 29:45, Al-Baqarah 2:152, Al-A'raf 7:205, Al-Jumu'ah 62:10, Al-Ahzaab 33:35, and Al-Ahzaab 33:41-42 [25]. Emphasizing the importance of verses that extoll the virtues of remembrance of Allah is a means of seeking closeness to Allah and finding peace.

Salah (Prayer) refers to the mandatory (five well-defined times a day) and voluntary prayers performed by Muslims. This establishes a direct connection with Allah by seeking peace, tranquility, and help while also expressing gratitude, invoking blessings, and purifying the heart [22, 23]. Evidence suggests the act of prayer improves the emotional management of personal problems [26], significantly improves depression and anxiety, increases daily spiritual experiences and optimism [27], and promotes a decrease in spiritual distress [28].

The recitation, the cycles of reflection, and the contemplation of the Holy Qur'an are considered as powerful means of finding solace and gaining strength to cope with life's challenges [22, 23]. Allah says in the Holy Qur'an: "*And We send down of the Qur'an that which is a healing and a mercy to those who believe (in Islamic Monotheism and act on it), and it increases the Zaalimoon (polytheists and wrongdoers) nothing but loss*" (Q Al-Israa 17:82). Research suggests that Qur'anic recitation can have a calming effect, reducing anxiety and stress levels in various settings [29], by inducing a relaxed cognitive and spiritual state [30, 31]. Owens et al. analyzed interventions using the Qur'an as a promoting factor for mental health [32]. The research indicated that prayer, supplications, recitation, reading, memorizing, and listening to the Qur'an reduced anxiety, depression, and stress, thus increasing the quality of life and coping. However, the authors concluded that Western countries often fail to utilize the Qur'an to promote culturally competent mental health care and support for the well-being of Muslim people.

The concepts of *sabr* (patience), acceptance, and trust in God (*tawakkul*) are integral to Islamic teachings. Muslims are encouraged to practice patience and acceptance in the face of hardship and challenges. Abu Yahya Suhaib bin Sinan, one of the companions of the Prophet (PBUH), reported that the Messenger of Allah (PBUH) said, "How wonderful is the case of a believer; there is good for him in everything, and this applies only to a believer. If prosperity attends him, he expresses gratitude to Allah and that is good for him; and if adversity befalls him, he endures it patiently and that is better for him" (Narrated by Muslim) [33]. Acceptance and putting one's trust in Allah involves two things: "depending on Allah and believing that He is the One Who causes measures to be effective" [34].

Inherent in Islamic teachings is *hilm* (forbearance), or being patient, calm, gentle, and forgiving in the face of adversity and challenges. Research suggests that forbearance can help Muslims cope by preventing anger, resentment, and revenge while also promoting acceptance, peace, harmony, and kindness [22]. One study showed the virtue of patience in decreasing symptoms of major depressive disorder and in dealing with life hardships including interpersonal and daily challenges [35].

Masjid (the mosque, the place of worship and prayers) serves as a gathering place for congregational prayers, religious activities, and community interactions. Muslims often seek solace by connecting with their fellow believers. The sense of belonging and support from fellow believers positively affects mental health and well-being [36]. *Istighfar* (Seeking forgiveness) and *tawbah* (repentance) are other coping mechanisms that provide a form of spiritual cleansing and relief from guilt so people can find peace and solace, thereby enabling individuals to make a fresh start. Divine forgiveness moderates the relationship between self-forgiveness and psychological distress, increasing coping and improving mental health and psychosocial wellbeing [37].

Conclusion

One aim of mental health care service delivery should be to support the development of culturally congruent health care for practicing Muslims globally. Western models of mental health care could utilize the Holy Qur'an for Muslim patients. This more closely relates to Islamic lifestyles through integrating teachings, beliefs, and practices into treatment planning, routine health care interventions, and delivery platforms. Using the Holy Qur'an has the potential to provide culturally competent mental health care for Muslim patients while simultaneously promoting positive coping, mental health, and well-being.

References

1. Ebrahimi, E. Spiritual health and psychosis in the light of Qur'an. *Journal of Arak University of Medical Sciences.* 2011;13(5):1–9.

2. Mahjoob, M., Nejati, J., Hosseini, A., & Bakhshani, N. M. The effect of Holy Qur'an voice on mental health. *Journal of Religion and Health.* 2016;55:38–42. http://dx.doi.org/10.1007/s10943-014-9821-7

3. Abu-Ras, W. & Abu-Bader, S. H. Risk factors for depression and post-traumatic stress disorder (PTSD): the case of Arab and Muslim Americans post–9/11. *Journal of Immigrant & Refugee Studies.* 2009;7(4):393–418. http://dx.doi.org/10.1080/15562940903379068

4. Heyman, J., Buchanan, R., Musgrave, B., & Menz, V. Social workers' attention to clients' spirituality: use of spiritual interventions in practice. *Arete.* 2006;30:78–89.

5. Hedayat-Diba, Z. Psychotherapy with Muslims. In: Richards, P. S. & Bergin, A. E., eds. *Handbook of Psychotherapy and Religious Diversity*. Washington, DC: American Psychological Association. 2000. 289–314.

6. Hodge, D. R. Social work and the house of Islam: orienting practitioners to the beliefs and values of Muslims in the United States. *Social Work*. 2005;50:162–73. https://doi.org/10.1093/sw/50.2.162

7. Mahmoud, V. African American Muslim families. In: McGoldrick, M., Giordano, J., & Pearce, J, K., eds. *Ethnicity and Family Therapy*. 2nd ed. New York: Guilford Press. 1996. 122–28.

8. Halligan, P. Caring for patients of Islamic denomination: critical care nurses' experiences in Saudi Arabia. *Journal of Clinical Nursing*. 2006;15(12):1565–73. https://doi.org/10.1111/j.1365-2702.2005.01525.x

9. Rassool, G. H. The Crescent and Islam: healing, nursing and the spiritual dimension. Some considerations towards an understanding of the Islamic perspectives on caring. *JAN*. 2000;32(6):1476–84. https://doi.org/10.1046/j.1365-2648.2000.01614.x

10. Pargament, K. I. *The Psychology of Religion and Coping: Theory, Research, and Practice*. New York: Guilford. 1997.

11. Pargament, K. I. & Ano, G. G. Spiritual resources and struggles in coping with medical illness. *Southern Medical Journal*. 2006;99:1161–62. https://doi.org/10.1097/01.smj.0000242847.40214.b6

12. McConnell, K. M., Pargament, K. I., Ellison, C. G., & Flannelly, K. J. Examining the links between spiritual struggles and symptoms of psychopathology in a national sample. *Journal of Clinical Psychology*. 2006;62:1469–84. https://doi.org/10.1002/jclp.20325

13. Engel, G. The need for a new medical model: a challenge for biomedicine. *Science*. 1977;196(4286):129–36. https://doi.org/10.1126/science.847460

14. Borrell-Carrió, F., Suchman, A. L., & Epstein, R. M. The biopsychosocial model 25 years later: principles, practice, and scientific inquiry. *Annals of Family Medicine*. 2004;2(6):576–82. https://doi.org/10.1370/afm.245

15. Abu-Raiya, H. & Pargament, K. I. Empirically based psychology of Islam: summary and critique of the literature. *Mental Health, Religion & Culture*. 2011;14(2):93–115. https://doi.org/10.1080/13674670903426482

16. Al-Sabwah, M. N. & Abdel-Khalek, A. M. Religiosity and death distress in Arabic college students. *Death Studies*. 2006;30(4):365–75. https://doi.org/10.1080/07481180600553435

17. Ai, A. L., Peterson, C., & Huang, B. The effect of religious-spiritual coping on positive attitudes of adult Muslim refugees from Kosovo and Bosnia. *The International Journal for the Psychology of Religion*. 2003;13(1):29–47. https://doi.org/10.1207/S15327582IJPR1301_04

18. Maqsood, R.W. *After Death Life! Thoughts to Alleviate the Grief of all Muslims Facing Death and Bereavement*. 4th ed. New Delhi: Good Word Books Ltd. 2002.

19. Sahih al-Bukhari. *Sahih al-Bukhari 3816*. In-book reference: Book 63, Hadith 41. Available from: https://sunnah.com/bukhari:3816

20. Subiyantoro, K., Primiana, I., Aldrin, S., & Febrian, H. R. The relationship between remembering God (*dhikr*) and stress prevention of life problem. *PalArch's Journal of Archaeology of Egypt/Egyptology*. 2020;17(7):4926–32.

21. Ibn Al-Qayyim. Cited in: Murad, K., ed. *In The Early Hours: Reflections on Spiritual and Self Development*. Markfield, UK: Revival Publications. 2004. 26.

22. Achour, M., Bensaid, B., & Nor, M. R. B. M. An Islamic perspective on coping with life stressors. *Applied Research in Quality of Life*. 2016;11:663–85. https://doi.org/10.1007/s11482-015-9389-8

23. Sultan, S. & Awad, N. 20 ways to cope with stress. [online]. Yaqeen Institute for Islamic Research. 2020 [Accessed July 4, 2023]. Video: 2:12 min. Available from: https://yaqeeninstitute.org/sarah-sultan/20-ways-to-cope-with-stress-animation

24. Sahih al-Bukhari. *Sahih al-Bukhari 7405*. In-book reference: Book 97, Hadith 34. Available from: https://sunnah.com/bukhari:7405

25. An-Nawawi, I. Cited in: Al-Nawawi, Y. S. Riyad as-Salihin: the meadows of the righteous. [online]. SunniPath: The Online Islamic Academy. n.d. [Accessed January 4, 2023]. Available from: https://web.archive.org/web/20110714123930/http://www.sunnipath.com/library/Hadith/H0004P0000.aspx

26. McCulloch, K. C. & Parks-Stamm, E. J. Reaching resolution: the effect of prayer on psychological perspective and emotional acceptance. *Psychology of Religion and Spirituality*. 2020;12 (2):254–59. https://doi.org/10.1037/rel0000234

27. Boelens, P. A., Reeves, R. R., Replogle, W. H., & Koenig, H. G. A randomized trial of the effect of prayer on depression and anxiety. *The International Journal of Psychiatry in Medicine*. 2009;39(4):377–92. https://doi.org/10.2190/PM.39.4.c

28. Miranda, T. P. S., Caldeira, S., de Oliveira, H. F., Iunes, D. H., Nogueira, D. A., Chaves, E. C. L., et al. Intercessory prayer on spiritual distress, spiritual coping, anxiety, depression and salivary amylase in breast cancer patients during radiotherapy: randomized clinical trial. *Journal of Religion and Health*. 2020;59 (1):365–80. https://doi.org/10.1007/s10943-019-00827-5

29. Ghiasi, A. & Keramat, A. The effect of listening to Holy Qur'an recitation on anxiety: a systematic review. *Iranian Journal of Nursing and Midwifery Research*. 2018;23(6):411–20. https://doi.org/10.4103/ijnmr.ijnmr_173_17

30. Kannan, M. A., Ab Aziz, N. A., Ab Rani, N. S., Abdullah, M. W., Rashil, M. H. M., Shab, M. S., et al. A review of the Holy Qur'an listening and its neural correlation for its potential as a psycho-spiritual therapy. *Heliyon*. 2022;8(12):e12308. https://doi.org/10.1016/j.heliyon.2022.e12308

31. Frih, B., Mkacher, W., Bouzguenda, A., Jaafar, H., Alkandari, S. A., Salah, B. Z., et al. Effects of listening to Holy Qur'an recitation and physical training on dialysis efficacy, functional capacity, and psychosocial outcomes in elderly patients undergoing haemodialysis. *Libyan Journal of Medicine*. 2017;12(1):1372032. https://doi.org/10.1080/19932820.2017.1372032

32. Owens, J., Rassool, G. H., Bernstein, J., Latif, S., & Aboul-Enein, B. H. Interventions using the Qur'an to promote mental health: a systematic scoping review. *Journal of Mental Health*. 2023;32(4):842–62. https://doi.org/10.1080/09638237.2023.2232449

33. Muslim. *Riyad as-Salihin 27*. In-book reference: Introduction, Hadith 27. Available from: https://sunnah.com/riyadussalihin:27

34. Islam Question & Answer. What is tawakkul? [online]. 2013 [Accessed January 4, 2023]. Available from: https://islamqa.info/en/answers/130499/putting-ones-trust-in-allah-and-taking-measures

35. Schnitker, S. A., Ro, D. B., Foster, J. D., Abernethy, A. D., Currier, J. M., Witvliet, C. V., et al. Patient patients: increased patience associated with decreased depressive symptoms in psychiatric treatment. *The Journal of Positive Psychology*. 2020;15(3):300–13. https://doi.org/10.1080/17439760.2019.1610482

36. Chen, Y., Harris, S. K., Worthington, E. L., Jr, & VanderWeele, T. J. Religiously or spiritually motivated forgiveness and subsequent health and well-being among young adults: an outcome-wide analysis. *The Journal of Positive Psychology*. 2019;14(5):649–58. https://doi.org/10.1080/17439760.2018.1519591

37. Fincham, F. D. & May, R. W. Self-forgiveness and well-being: does divine forgiveness matter? *The Journal of Positive Psychology*. 2019;14(6):854–59. https://doi.org/10.1080/17439760.2019.1579361

Maternal and Child Health: An Islamic Perspective

Fatmah Almoayad

Introduction

Maternal and child health (MCH) focuses on ensuring women's, children's, and families' well-being [1, 2]. It incorporates societal efforts to facilitate healthy pregnancies, childbirth, and child development. Recognized globally as a key investment, MCH is reflected in the United Nation's Sustainable Development Goals (SDGs) [3]. Islamic scriptures emphasize MCH in the Holy Qur'an and Prophetic Hadith, offering insights into Islam's role in maternal and child welfare. This chapter explores these Islamic teachings, stressing social support, nutrition, and education, and demonstrates their alignment with global initiatives such as the United Nations Convention on the Rights of the Child (UNCRC).

Pregnancy

The Qur'an describes the process of fetal development in several verses. In Q Al-Hajj 22:5 it states,

> O mankind! If ye have any doubt about the Resurrection, (Consider) that We created you Out of dust, then out of Sperm, then out of a leech like Clot, then out a morsel Of flesh, partly formed And partly unformed, in order That We may manifest (Our power) to you; And We cause whom We will To rest in the wombs For an appointed term, Then do We bring you out As babes, then (foster you) That ye may reach your age Of full strength; and some Of you are called to die, And some are sent back To the feeblest old age, So that they know nothing After having known (much).

In Q Al-Mu'minun 23:12–15, it further states,

> Man We did create From a quintessence (of clay); Then We placed him As (a drop of) sperm In a place of rest, Firmly fixed; Then We made the sperm Into a clot of congealed blood; Then of that clot We made A (foetus) lump; then We Made out of that lump Bones and clothed the bones With flesh; then We developed Out of it another creature. So blessed be God, The Best to create!

Islam emphasizes social support for women during pregnancy and obligates the father of the offspring to take financial care of the pregnant or breastfeeding woman, even if divorced, as stated in Q Yusuf 12:6:

> Let the women live (In 'iddat) in the same Style as ye live, According to your means: Annoy them not, so as To restrict them. And if they carry (life In their wombs), then Spend (your substance) on them Until they deliver Their burden: and if They suckle your (offspring), Give them their recompense: And take mutual counsel Together, according to What is just and reasonable.

The care for a mother is not limited to the father of the offspring but extends to the offspring beyond the years of pregnancy and breastfeeding, as stated in Q Al-Ahqaaf 46:15, "*We have enjoined on man Kindness to his parents: In pain did his mother Bear him, and in pain Did she give him birth,*" and in Q Luqmaan 31:14, "*And We have enjoined on man (To be good) to his parents: In travail upon travail Did his mother bear him, And in years twain Was his weaning: (hear The command), 'Show gratitude To Me and to thy parents: To Me is (thy final) Goal'*". This support is of high importance to pregnant women's health and well-being in light of the existing evidence linking the lack of social support with pregnancy, mental health problems, and self-harm [4].

In addition, Islam advises against burdening people beyond their abilities, as stated in Q Al-Baqarah 2:286: "*On no soul doth God place a burden greater than it can bear.*" The Prophet (PBUH) also said, "If I command you to do a thing, then do as much of it as you can" [5, 6]. Thus, pregnant women are permitted to adapt their religious practices according to their physical abilities. The two most distinct examples are, first, exceptions from Ramadan fasting, as stated in Q Al-Baqarah 2:184: "*(Fasting) for a fixed number of days; but if any of you is ill or on a journey the prescribed number (should be made up) from days later. For those who can do it (with hardship) is a ransom the feeding of one that is indigent,*" and, second, allowing for changes in prayer positions, as Prophet Muhammad (PBUH) said: "Pray standing, and if you cannot, then sitting down, and if you cannot, then lying on your side" [7] and "God has remitted half the prayer to the traveler, and fasting to the traveler, the woman who is suckling an infant and the woman who is pregnant" [8]. Overall, Islam emphasizes the importance of supporting pregnant women both socially and financially and provides clear guidance on not burdening individuals beyond their abilities. This support is crucial for the health and well-being of pregnant women and their offspring.

All of this indicates that Islam stresses the multifaceted support for pregnant women. The Holy Qur'an outlines the process of fetal development and emphasizes the importance of paternal care and allowances for mothers-to-be. Pregnant women are granted allowances, such as exemption from fasting during Ramadan and adjustments in prayer positions, ensuring they are not burdened beyond their capacity. This approach fosters the health and well-being of pregnant women and their offspring.

Breastfeeding

Breastfeeding is one of the most important nutritional concerns promoted by the WHO to achieve the SDGs [9]. The importance of breastfeeding is promoted for its multiple levels of benefits, starting with the prevention of many noncommunicable diseases both in childhood and later in life. Additionally, there are health benefits for the breastfeeding mother, such as the prevention of breast cancer [10]. In Islam, breastfeeding is a right of the child that is endorsed in many verses of the Holy Qur'an, including Q Al-Baqarah 2:233:

> The mothers shall give suck to their offspring for two whole years if the father desires to complete the term. But he shall bear the cost of their food and clothing on equitable terms. No soul shall have a burden laid on it greater than it can bear. No mother shall be treated unfairly on account of her child nor father on account of his child. An heir shall be chargeable in the same way if they both decide on weaning by mutual consent and after due consultation there is no blame on them. If ye decide on a foster-mother for your offspring there is no blame

on you provided ye pay (the mother) what ye offered on equitable terms. But fear God and know that God sees well what ye do.

This verse reserves the rights of both the child and the mother. The mother should not be burdened beyond what she can bear, and fathers are instructed to provide breastfeeding mothers with financial support and fair treatment, even in the case of a divorce [11]. The literature has shown that paternal support and other family members' support of breastfeeding is crucial [12].

If the mother is unable to breastfeed, Islam maintains the infant's right to breastfeeding by allowing the father to contract with a wet nurse upon the agreement of both parents [11]. A wet nurse, whether hired or donated to breastfeed an infant, has a lifelong connection with the nursed infant called "milk kinship," by which the breastfeeding mother and her husband are considered parents of that infant and their children the infant's siblings [13]. This is mentioned in Q An-Nisa 4:23:

Forbidden to you are your mothers and your daughters and your sisters and your paternal aunts and your maternal aunts and brothers' daughters and sisters' daughters and your mothers that have suckled you and your foster-sisters and mothers of your wives and your step-daughters who are in your guardianship, (born) of your wives to whom you have gone in, but if you have not gone into them, there is no blame on you (in marrying them), and the wives of your sons who are of your own loins and that you should have two sisters together, except what has already passed; surely Allah is Forgiving, Merciful.

This kinship requires Muslim mothers to know who they breastfeed and who wet-nurses their children, which prevents them from engaging in anonymous milk donation [14].

The recommended period of breastfeeding as mentioned in the Holy Qur'an is up to two years [11]. This is mentioned in several verses such as Q Luqmaan 31:14: "*And in years twain was his weaning.*" In Q Al-Ahqaaf 46:15 it states, "*The carrying of the (child) To his weaning is (A period of) thirty months,*" and in Q Al-Baqarah 2:233, "*The mothers shall give suck to their offspring for two whole years.*" This two-year recommendation is similar to the two years of breastfeeding recommended by the WHO [15]. In conclusion, breastfeeding is highly emphasized in Islam as a right of the child, with clear guidance on the length of the recommended period and the father's responsibilities to provide financial support. This aligns with the WHO's promotion of breastfeeding as a key component in achieving the SDGs and the numerous health benefits it provides for both the mother and child.

Child Welfare

The UNCRC, a legally binding document, protects children's welfare [16]. Article 6 acknowledges every child's right to life and stresses the importance of protecting and promoting the survival and development of every child. The Qur'an aligns with this, prohibiting child killing and sex discrimination. The Qur'an emphasizes the right to life, countering pre-Islamic practices of child-killing due to poverty or honor preservation [16]. Q Al-Kahf 18:46 indicates the blessing of having children: "*Wealth and children are the adornment of this worldly life.*" Q Ash-Shura 42:49–50 highlights that having children and deciding their sex is God's will for reasons and wisdom beyond humans: "*To God belongs the dominion of the heavens and the earth. He creates what He wills (And plans). He bestows (Children) male or female According to His Will (and Plan), Or He bestows both males And females, and He leaves Barren whom He will: For He is full Of knowledge and power"* Other verses clearly prohibit the harming and killing of infants, such as Q Al-An'am 6:151: *"Say to them: 'Come, let me recite what your Lord has laid down to you: that you associate nothing with Him; and do good to your parents; and do not slay your children out of fear of poverty."* In Q Al-A'raf 7:31, it states, *"O children of Adam, take your adornment [i.e., wear your clothing] at every masjid, and eat and drink, but be not excessive. Indeed, He likes not those who commit excess."* In addition, Q At-Takweer 81:8–9 describes the following: *"When the female (infant), Buried alive, is questioned – For what crime She was killed."*

The Qur'an not only prohibits the act of killing female infants but also condemns the behavior of discrimination against girls, as in Q An-Nahl 16:58–59: *"When news is brought to one of them, of (the birth Of) a female (child), his face Darkens, and he is filled With inward grief! With shame does he hide Himself from his people, Because of the bad news He has had! Shall he retain it on (sufferance and) contempt, Or bury it in the dust? Ah! what an evil (choice) They decide on?"* This aligns with The UNCRC which emphasized many articles on children's rights without distinction of sex [16].

The UNCRC, in Articles 7 and 8, upholds a child's right to preserve their identity, including their name and family connections [16]. These rights are also reserved in Islam in which every child has the right of legitimacy and belonging to their families [17]. This right is initially reserved by the protection of lineage and the prohibition of fornication and having children outside marriage [18]. Q Al-Ahzaab 33:5 states,

> Call them by [the names of] their fathers; it is more just in the sight of Allah. But if you do not know their fathers – then they are [still] your brothers in religion and those entrusted to you. And there is no blame upon you for that in which you have erred but [only for] what your hearts intended. And ever is Allah Forgiving and Merciful.

The naming of the child is a reserved right for the child as the Prophet Muhammad (PBUH) guided. Moreover, the Prophet (PBUH) instructed the parents to choose a good name for their children as he said, "On the Day of Resurrection you will be called by your names and by your father's names, so give yourselves good names" [19].

The UNCRC's Article 28 emphasizes education as an essential aspect of child welfare [16]. Education is considered a significant priority in Islam, and it has always emphasized the importance of acquiring knowledge and education. The very first revelation of the Qur'an to Prophet Muhammad (PBUH) was Q Al-Alaq 96:1–5: *"Read! In the Name of your Lord, Who has created (all that exists), He has created man from a clot (a piece of thick coagulated blood), Read! And your Lord is the Most Generous, Who has taught (the writing) by the pen, He has taught man that which he knew not."* This illustrates the high importance given to education in Islam. Furthermore, Prophet Muhammad (PBUH) is reported to have said, "Seeking knowledge is an obligation upon every Muslim" [20].

The welfare of children is highly valued in both Islam and the UNCRC. The Qur'anic verses emphasize the protection of the child's right to life and the importance of education, while the convention protects the child's right to identity, non-discrimination, and education. These protections should ensure children are treated with respect and dignity and are given the necessary tools to grow and thrive in a supportive environment.

Conclusion

In conclusion, this chapter provided a comprehensive overview of Islamic teachings on pregnancy, breastfeeding, and child welfare, demonstrating the religion's emphasis on the well-being of mothers and children. It explored Qur'anic verses and Hadiths that underline the importance of social support, nutrition, and education in the lives of mothers and children. Islamic teachings provide a solid foundation for promoting a supportive, nurturing, and civic environment for mothers and children. Islam emphasizes the significance of social support and financial assistance during pregnancy, encourages breastfeeding, and emphasizes child welfare through the protection of life, identity, and education. These principles align with and contribute to global efforts to improve maternal and child health and could serve as culturally congruent approaches for maternal/child health educators and practitioners in Muslim-majority communities.

References

1. Ki-Moon, B. *Global Strategy for Women's and Children's Health*. New York: United Nations. 2010.

2. Lu, M. C. The future of maternal and child health. *Maternal and Child Health Journal*. 2019;23(1):1–7. https://doi.org/10.1007/s10995-018-2643-6

3. Mohammed, A. J. A call to action: improving women's, children's, and adolescents' health in the Muslim world. *The Lancet*. 2018;391(10129):1458–60. https://doi.org/10.1016/S0140-6736(18)30182-X

4. Bedaso, A., Adams, J., Peng, W., & Sibbritt, D. The relationship between social support and mental health problems during pregnancy: a systematic review and meta-analysis. *Reproductive Health*. 2021;18(1):162. https://doi.org/10.1186/s12978-021-01209-5

5. Sahih Muslim. *Sahih Muslim 1337*. In-book reference: Book 15, Hadith 461. Available from: https://sunnah.com/muslim:1337

6. Sahih al-Bukhari. *Sahih al-Bukhari 7288*. In-book reference: Book 96, Hadith 19. Available from: https://sunnah.com/bukhari:7288

7. Sahih al-Bukhari. *Sahih al-Bukhari 1117*. In-book reference: Book 18, Hadith 37. Available from: https://sunnah.com/bukhari:1117

8. Sunan Abi Dawud. *Sunan Abi Dawud 2408*. In-book reference: Book 14, Hadith 96. Available from: https://sunnah.com/abudawud:2408

9. World Health Organization. *The Best Start in Life: Breastfeeding for the Prevention of Noncommunicable Diseases and the Achievement of the Sustainable Development Goals in the WHO European Region*. Copenhagen: World Health Organization Regional Office for Europe. 2020.

10. Slusser, W. Breastfeeding and maternal and infant health outcomes in developed countries. *AAP Grand Rounds*. 2007;18(2):15–16. https://doi.org/10.1542/gr.18-2-15

11. Bensaid, B. Breastfeeding as a fundamental Islamic human right. *Journal of Religion and Health*. 2021;60(1):362–73. https://doi.org/10.1007/s10943-019-00835-5

12. Clifford, J. & McIntyre, E. Who supports breastfeeding? *Breastfeeding Review*. 2008;16(2):9–19.

13. Zaidi, F. Challenges and practices in infant feeding in Islam. *British Journal of Midwifery*. 2014;22(3):167–72. https://doi.org/10.12968/bjom.2014.22.3.167

14. Subudhi, S. & Sriraman, N. Islamic beliefs about milk kinship and donor human milk in the United States. *Pediatrics*. 2021;147(2):e20200441. https://doi.org/10.1542/peds.2020-0441

15. World Health Organization. *Global Strategy for Infant and Young Child Feeding*. Geneva: World Health Organization. 2003.

16. UNICEF. Convention on the Rights of the Child. [online]. 1989 [Accessed March 4, 2023]. Available from: www.unicef.org/child-rights-convention/convention-text

17. Omran, A. R. Children's rights in Islam from the Qur'an and Sunnah. *Population Sciences*. 1990;9:77–88.

18. Ihwani, S. S., Muhtar, A., Musa, N., Yaakub, A., Mohamad, A. M., Hehsan, A., et al. An overview of sex education: comparison between Islam and Western perspectives. *Al-Qanatir: International Journal of Islamic Studies*. 2017;8 (4):43–51.

19. Sunan Abi Dawud. *Sunan Abi Dawud 4948*. In-book reference: Book 43, Hadith 176. Available from: https://sunnah.com/abudawud:4948

20. Sunan Ibn Majah. *Sunan Ibn Majah 224*. In-book reference: Introduction, Hadith 224. Available from: https://sunnah.com/ibnmajah:224

Chapter 5

Immunization and Islamic Guidance

Janine Owens

Introduction

Islam entrusts Muslims with caring for their bodies by protecting and maintaining them. The holistic approach to health taken by Islam allows cures from both spiritual means and medical science because Allah creates both the disease and treatment, and, in the case of medical science, Allah works through the health care professional. Narrated by Abu Huraira, the Prophet (PBUH) said, "There is no disease that Allah has created, except that He has also created its treatment" [1]. Islamic religious law (Sharia) discusses the preservation and protection of the human body throughout the life course. This includes parents paying attention to the physical health and well-being of their children by meeting their health needs. Sharia regulates many aspects of Muslim life, including the protection of children, and in return it reinforces the legal duty of children to support their parents in sickness and old age. One example of the impact of Sharia on increased child protection is its introduction in Nigeria, which increased the incidence of child vaccination by 20% and extended breastfeeding by two months on average [2].

In Islam, the parents as guardians are responsible for ensuring that they meet their children's basic care needs.

The Prophet Muhammad (PBUH) said, "The man is a guardian of his family; the lady is a guardian and is responsible for her husband's house and his offspring" [3]. Neglecting a child's basic needs would be a violation of Islamic teachings and law. The needs of a child, including guidance on nutrition and feeding, are clearly cited in the Holy Qur'an: "*Mothers may nurse [i.e., breastfeed] their children two complete years for whoever wishes to complete the nursing [period]*" (Q Al-Baqarah 2:233). However, if breastfeeding is not possible, it is permissible to use alternatives such as a wet nurse or specifically designed baby formula to meet the nutritional needs of the child while fulfilling the obligation of parents as protectors. Other health and spiritual guidance as well as legislation in Sharia prohibits abandonment, neglect, and harm. Vaccination is included under the role of protecting the health of the child, and the parent is obligated to use this treatment through Sharia and Islamic teachings. Vaccination is also a way of protecting populations from the transmission of communicable diseases.

The teachings of Prophet Muhammad (PBUH) advise on the concept of quarantine, instructing his companions to adhere to preventive behaviors: "If you hear about it (an outbreak of plague) in a land, do not go to it; but if the plague breaks out in a country where you are staying, do not run away from it" [4]. The reason for quarantine is to prevent the spread of disease within and between populations. At the time of Allah's Messenger (PBUH), vaccination had not been developed, and therefore quarantine was the most effective alternative.

Challenges to Vaccine Uptake for Muslims

One challenge to vaccine uptake for Muslims is the concept that substances, which are impure (*naajis*) or forbidden (*haram*), should not enter the body. The Holy Qur'an states, "Forbidden to you are carrion, blood, and swine; what is slaughtered in the name of any other than Allah ... and intoxicants" (Q Al-Ma'idah 5:3, 91). In some countries, parents believe that porcine (swine) derivatives (such as trypsin and gelatin) contaminate vaccines, making them *haram* for Muslims [5, 6, 7]. However, the World Health Organization (WHO) for the Eastern Mediterranean reported the alteration of porcine sources during the process of vaccine development and production, which changes them into another substance without similarity to the original source [8, 9]. Within Islam, the process of perfect change (*Istihaalah*) means that a substance can change into another, exhibiting different characteristics. Therefore, an impure substance may change into a pure substance, or a *haram* substance may change into one that is permissible according to Sharia. Furthermore, in 2003, the European Council of Fatwa and Research ruled that if the amount of porcine sources is insignificant or almost negligible in any vaccine, then it is too small to be of importance or to exert any effect [10].

Another challenge to vaccine uptake is misinformation from social media, mass media, and, in some cases, from community leaders. For example, Millennium Development Goal (MDG) 4 included the reduction of childhood mortality by two-thirds by 2015 [11] and the eradication of polio by 2005, now moved to 2026, as part of the Global Polio Eradication Initiative (GPEI) [12]. In 2003, polio was endemic in seven countries, one of which was Nigeria. In 2023, it is only in two: Pakistan and Afghanistan [12]. In 2003, Muslim and political leaders in northern Nigeria placed the MDG 4 and the aims of the GPEI under threat by bringing the polio immunization campaign to a standstill [13]. This emerged from misinformation that the West deliberately contaminated the vaccines with anti-fertility agents and HIV in a plot to reduce the global Muslim population. A resolution occurred when Nigerian religious leaders received assurance about vaccine safety and subsequently confirmed its acceptability to the communities [13]. This had happened previously in Cameroon [14] and Uganda [15], but polio was also not a priority for the local communities there who were worried about malaria and were dissatisfied with the lack of primary health care.

Other challenges to vaccine uptake faced by Muslims are varied. For example, there is the issue of perceived discrimination and deprivation experienced by Muslim populations living in segregated neighborhoods in Aligarh - Utter Pradesh state in India [16]. These neighborhoods exhibit a lack of infrastructure development; poor sanitation, housing, and education; a lack of inclusive health systems; and an overall lack of public health awareness [16]. This situation led to distrust in the government and GPEI workers, the spread of misinformation, social resistance to vaccine uptake, higher transmission rates, and a rise in polio disparity [16]. To address the problem, UNICEF reached out to these communities and engaged with local leaders while also providing basic health provisions to illustrate the consideration of their health needs [16, 17, 18].

A recent challenge in 2021 was the introduction of COVID-19 vaccinations during Ramadan (Islamic month of fasting) when Muslims are required to refrain from anything entering the body during fasting hours. To address the potential for vaccine hesitancy, Muslim scholars issued a ruling advising that accepting the COVID-19 vaccination during Ramadan did not invalidate the fast because the delivery is through injection and not via the mouth or nose [19].

Other challenges revolve around the structure of Western health services. One example of poor vaccine uptake among Lebanese immigrant Muslims emerged from Australia [19]. In this study, Muslim patients valued information and the discussions they had with nurses, but cultural attitudes regarding the roles of nurses and medical staff coupled with the lack of awareness from health professionals about Lebanese Muslim cultural and religious beliefs made health protection challenging [20]. This is apparent in more recent studies discussing health care staff, implicit bias (unconscious attitudes and stereotyping), and a lack of consideration for Muslim religious beliefs [21, 22].

There is also the issue of the religious health fatalism belief where one reason for parents' refusal of vaccination for their children in Malaysia was that during the creation of humans God bestowed upon them an immune system to fight against disease; therefore, vaccines were unnecessary [23]. These parents interpreted Islamic teachings more fundamentally, failing to consider the majority rulings about benefit over risk of harm emerging from Islamic scholars and jurisprudence based on the best interests of the child. Higher religious health fatalism beliefs in other studies lowered the intention to receive the COVID-19 vaccination [24, 25].

Participation in human papillomavirus (HPV) vaccination is low in some Muslim populations. The detection rate of HPV is 99% in cervical cancers and the high-risk oncogenic HPV subtypes. Vaccination protects against the virus by preventing persistent infection with one of the 15 HPV subtypes [26]. In the Netherlands, cervical cancer is the second most common cancer among Muslim Somali women [27]. Reasons for not vaccinating include the belief that not having sex before marriage is a protective factor and therefore vaccination is not relevant to them. Another reason is the Dutch language barrier, because young Dutch-speaking Somali girls would need to translate for their mothers about a subject viewed as inappropriate for discussion [27]. There is also the lack of culturally informed information at schools, mistrust in Dutch health care and the government, misinformation, and the taboo around discussing cancer with the associated belief that it was God's will, returning to religious health fatalism [23–25, 27].

Parents who believed that the benefits of vaccination outweighed the risks appeared in a study on Arab Israeli Muslims and the vaccination of their children against influenza [28]. This particular study indicated that community nurses and doctors played a role in parents' decision-making by raising awareness of the risks of seasonal influenza and the benefits of vaccination. Parents were also younger and had fewer children, suggesting that this gave them more time to consider the benefits and risks when deciding about vaccination.

Public Health and Vaccination of Muslims

The evidence suggests that while Islamic teachings are a protective factor they can simultaneously be a barrier to health protection and prevention because of the way people interpret the teachings alongside the influence of cultural beliefs and attitudes.

To respond to parental concerns about immunization safety, health care professionals and nongovernmental organizations (NGOs) working with Muslim parents need training on how to respond, what to expect, and what to do [20]. Non-Muslim NGOs and health care professionals need to develop an awareness of Islamic teachings and cultural competence with the understanding that Muslim communities are diverse and culture may influence the interpretation of Islamic teachings [23, 24, 25].

In a study on Arab Israeli Muslims, the evidence suggested that interventions for immunization should begin on the micro (patient) level with the parent–health care professional encounter and the development of a relationship of mutual trust and respect [28]. This relationship is important when making choices and decisions about immunization and minimizes issues such as distrust that were mentioned in other studies [5, 11, 13–15, 26].

Some studies with Muslim communities in India use intensive social mobilization techniques, such as inviting trusted leaders and respected women in the communities to carry out awareness-raising and trust-building activities, thereby achieving significant increases in vaccination [29]. Social mobilization involves engaging governments, communities, traditional and opinion leaders, NGOs, and health care professionals in solving a common health problem. The partnerships between these different groups assist in developing solutions, often through awareness-raising campaigns. Above all, the focus is participatory and on communities developing organic, culturally congruent solutions rather than having solutions imposed upon them.

For example, studies on immunization against rotavirus in Indonesia utilize Muslim religious leaders who are willing to provide support in the introduction of vaccines by advocating for their safety and using Islamic teachings to encourage community engagement [30]. Other studies argue that religious leaders feel their role extends past the post-introduction period, including advocacy for immunization prior to the introduction of a new vaccine and during implementation, and that they are an integral part of the ongoing program [31]. Globally, the WHO SAGE Vaccine Hesitancy Working Group acknowledges the influence of community and religious leaders on vaccine acceptance and recognizes the positive effects of interventions engaging religious or other influential leaders to promote vaccination in the community [32, 33].

Conclusion

Islamic teachings promote the protection of populations and the role of parents as protectors of their children, and immunization is one way of protecting populations and children from harm. The challenges of immunizing Muslim populations are numerous. The evidence does, however, underline the importance of engaging with Muslim communities, their religious leaders, and opinion leaders through discussion, education, and social mobilization. Public health aims to develop culturally competent health care professionals who can develop trusting relationships with Muslim communities. There is also a need among Muslim populations to promote awareness about the hazards of not immunizing, to prevent the spread of misinformation, to address religious concerns about vaccines being *haram*, and to encourage communities to play an active role in vaccine promotion. This approach is more successful when communities have lower competing demands on their resources and when governments address issues like lack of education or poor housing and sanitation and develop equitable access to employment and health care.

References

1. Sahih al-Bukhari. *Sahih al-Bukhari 5678.* In-book reference: Book 76, Hadith 1. Available from: https://sunnah.com/bukhari:5678

2. Alfano, M. Islamic law and investments in children: evidence from the Sharia introduction in Nigeria. *Journal of Health Economics.* 2022;85:102260. https://doi.org/10.1016/j.jhealeco.2022.102660

3. Sahih al-Bukhari. *Sahih al-Bukhari 5200.* In-book reference: Book 67, Hadith 134. Available from: https://sunnah.com/bukhari:5200

4. Sahih al-Bukhari. *Sahih al-Bukhari 5729.* In-book reference: Book 76, Hadith 44. Available from: https://sunnah.com/bukhari:5729

5. Ahmed, A., Lee, K. S., Bukhsh, A., Al-Worafi, Y. M., Sarker, M. M. R., Ming, L. C., et al. Outbreak of vaccine-preventable diseases in Muslim majority countries. *Journal of Infection and Public Health.* 2018;11(2):153–55. https://doi.org/10.1016/j.jiph.2017.09.007

6. Harjaningrum, A. T., Kartasasmita, C., Orne-Gliemann, J., Jutand, M. A., Goujon, N., & Koeck, J. L. A qualitative study on knowledge, perceptions, and attitudes of mothers and health care providers toward pneumococcal conjugate vaccine in Bandung, West Java, Indonesia. *Vaccine.* 2013;31(11):1516–22. https://doi.org/10.1016/j.vaccine.2013.01.007

7. Wong, L. P. & Sam, I. C. Factors influencing the uptake of 2009 H1N1 influenza vaccine in a multi-ethnic Asian population. *Vaccine.* 2010;28(28):4499–505. https://doi.org/10.1016/j.vaccine.2010.04.043

8. Gezairy, H. A. WHO letter reports on Islamic Legal Scholars' verdict on the medicinal use of gelatin derived from pork products. Cairo: World Health Organization (WHO) for the Eastern Mediterranean. 2001.

9. World Health Organization Regional Office for the Eastern Mediterranean. *Statement Arising From a Seminar Held by the Islamic Organization for Medical Sciences on "The Judicially Prohibited and Impure Substances in Foodstuff and Drugs."* 2001. Available from: www.immunize.org/concerns/porcine.pdf

10. European Council of Fatwa and Research. Eleventh regular session of the European Council of Fatwa and Research. Stockholm: European Council of Fatwa and Research. 2003.

11. World Health Organization. Millennium development goals. [online]. 2018 [Accessed March 2, 2023]. Available from: https://www.who.int/news-room/fact-sheets/detail/millennium-development-goals-(mdgs)

12. World Health Organization. *Polio Eradication Strategy 2022–2026: Delivering on a Promise.* Geneva: World Health Organization. 2021.

13. Yahya, M. Polio vaccines: "no thank you!" barriers to polio eradication in northern Nigeria. *African Affairs.* 2007;106(423):185–204. https://doi.org/10.1093/afraf/adm016

14. Ghinai, I., Willott, C., Dadari, I., & Larson, H. J. Listening to the rumours: what the northern Nigeria polio vaccine boycott can tell us ten years on. *Global Public Health.* 2013;8(10):1138–50. https://doi.org/10.1080/17441692.2013.859720

15. Feldman-Savelsberg, P., Ndonko, F. T., & Schmidt-Ehry, B. Sterilizing vaccines or the politics of the womb: retrospective study of a rumor in Cameroon. *Medical Anthropology Quarterly.* 2000;14(2):159–79. https://doi.org/10.1525/maq.2000.14.2.159

16. UNICEF Eastern and Southern Africa Regional Office. *Combating Antivaccination Rumours: Lessons Learned from Case Studies in East Africa.* 2002. Available from: www.poliokit.org/sites/default/files/migrate/2013_UNICEF_ESARO-_Lessons_learned_East_Africa_combatting_rumours.pdf

17. Hussain, R. S., McGarvey, S. T., & Fruzzetti, L. M. Partition and

poliomyelitis: an investigation of the polio disparity affecting Muslims during India's eradication program. *PLoS ONE.* 2015;10(3):e0115628. https://doi.org/10.1371/journal.pone.0115628

18. Ansari, M. A., Khan, Z., Mehnaz, S., Shah, M. S., Abedi, A. J., & Ahmad, A. L. Role of social mobilization in tackling the resistance to polio eradication program in underserved communities of Aligarh, India. *WHO-SEAJPH.* 2014;3(2):23–29. https://doi.org/10.3329/seajph.v3i2.20035

19. UNICEF. Ramadan 2021: Staying safe and getting vaccinated for COVID-19. [online]. 2021 [Accessed March 3, 2023]. Available from: https://www.unicef.org/rosa/stories/ramadan-2021-staying-safe-and-getting-vaccinated-covid-19

20. Brooke, D. & Omeri, A. Beliefs about childhood immunisation among Lebanese Muslim immigrants in Australia. *Journal of Transcultural Nursing.* 1999;10(3):229–36. https://doi.org/10.1177/104365969901000314

21. Alsuwaidi, A. L., Al-Karim Hammad, H. A., Elbarazi, I., & Sheek-Hussain, M. Vaccine hesitancy within the Muslim community: Islamic faith and public health perspectives. *Human Vaccines & Immunotherapeutics.* 2023;19(1):2190716. https://doi.org/10.1080/21645515.2023.2190716

22. Neggaz, M. Vaccine uptake and hesitancy among American Muslims. [online]. ISPU. 2021 [Accessed March 3, 2023]. Available from: www.ispu.org/vaccine-uptake-and-hesitancy/

23. Rumetta, J., Abdul-Hadi, H., & Lee, Y. K. A qualitative study on parents' reasons and recommendations for childhood vaccination refusal in Malaysia. *Journal of Infection and Public Health.* 2020;13 (2):199–203. https://doi.org/10.1016/j.jiph.2019.07.027

24. Wong, L. P., Alias, H., Megat Hashim, M. M. A. A., Lee, H. Y., AbuBakar, S., Chung, I., et al. Acceptability for COVID-19 vaccination: perspectives from Muslims. *Human Vaccines & Immunotherapeutics.* 2022;18(5):2045855. https://doi.org/10.1080/21645515.2022.2045855

25. Murakami, H., Kobayashi, M., Hachiya, M., Khan, Z. S., Hassan, S. Q., & Sakurada, S. Refusal of oral polio vaccine in northwestern Pakistan: a qualitative and quantitative study. *Vaccine.* 2014;32 (12):1382–87. https://doi.org/10.1016/j.vaccine.2014.01.018

26. Cutts, F. T., Franceschi, S., Goldie, S., Castellsague, X., de Sanjose, S., Garnett, G., et al. Human papillomavirus and HPV vaccines: a review. *Bulletin of the World Health Organization.* 2007;85(9):719–26. https://doi.org/10.2471/blt.06.038414

27. Salad, J., Verdonk, P., de Boer, F., & Abma, T. A. "A Somali girl is Muslim and does not have premarital sex. Is vaccination really necessary?" A qualitative study into the perceptions of Somali women in the Netherlands about the prevention of cervical cancer. *International Journal for Equity in Health.* 2015;14:68. https://doi.org/10.1186/s12939-015-0198-3

28. Ben Natan, M., Kabha, S., Yehia, M., & Hamza, O. Factors that influence Israeli Muslim Arab parents' intention to vaccinate their children against influenza. *Journal of Pediatric Nursing.* 2016;31 (3):293–98. https://doi.org/10.1016/j.pedn.2015.12.014

29. Choudhary, M., Solomon, R., Awale, J., Dey, R., Singh, J. P., & Weiss, W. Significance of a social mobilization intervention for engaging communities in polio vaccination campaigns: evidence from CORE Group Polio Project, Uttar Pradesh, India. *Journal of Global Health.* 2021;10(11):07011. https://doi.org/10.7189/jogh.11.07011

30. Padmawati, R. S., Heywood, A., Sitaresmi, M. N., Atthobari, J., MacIntyre, C. R., Soenarto, Y., et al. Religious and community leaders' acceptance of rotavirus vaccine introduction in Yogyakarta, Indonesia: a qualitative study. *BMC Public Health.* 2019;19 (1):368. https://doi.org/10.1186/s12889-019-6706-4

31. Paterson, P. & Larson, H. J. The role of publics in the introduction of new vaccines. *Health Policy and Planning.*

2012;27(Suppl 2):ii77–79. https://doi.org/10.1093/heapol/czs038

32. The Working Group. *Report of the SAGE Working Group on Vaccine Hesitancy.* 2014. Available from: www.asset-scienceinsociety.eu/sites/default/files/sage_working_group_revised_report_vaccine_hesitancy.pdf

33. Jarrett, C., Wilson, R., O'Leary, M., Eckersberger, E., Larson, H. J., & The SAGE Working Group on Vaccine Hesitancy. Strategies for addressing vaccine hesitancy: a systematic review. *Vaccine.* 2015;33(34):4180–90. https://doi.org/10.1016/j.vaccine.2015.04.040

Sexual and Reproductive Health: An Islamic Perspective

Noura Alomair, Nour Horanieh, Samah Alageel

Sex and Sexuality under Islamic Law

Marriage or *nikah* in Islam is the sacred union of a man and a woman. Marriage in Islam is thought to complete half of one's faith and religious obligations [1]. Sexual relations are permissible within marriage. Sexual intercourse is viewed as a way for couples to connect and strengthen their relationship. Polygamy is permissible in Islam, where men are allowed to marry up to four women at the same time, while Muslim women can only marry one man at a time. However, there is no limit to how many husbands a woman can marry throughout her lifetime [2]. As for interfaith marriages, Muslim women can only marry Muslim men, whereas Muslim men are allowed to marry women from the Muslim, Christian, or Jewish faiths [3].

Sex outside of a lawful marriage is called *zina* and is considered forbidden under Islamic law and is described as a *fahisha* or obscenity. The same word is used to describe sodomy or anal sex, which is forbidden in Islam. Homosexuality is also forbidden in Islam and punishable under Islamic law [4].

Divorce, or *talaq*, is permitted in Islam [5, 6]. A nonpregnant woman must remain single for three months after the divorce, a period called *iddah*, before being allowed to marry another man. If the woman wants a divorce, she needs to ask her husband to divorce her; if he refuses, she must file a case in court. For this form of divorce, called *khul'* and which requires a judge's approval, the woman must provide the judge with legitimate reasons for divorce and give back her dowry [6]. The *iddah* in this form of divorce is one month. If a woman loses her husband to death, her *iddah* is 4 months and 10 days. However, if a woman is pregnant, all forms of *iddah* would extend until she gives birth to the child to ensure the lineage of children is known. Men do not observe *iddahs* upon the divorce or death of a wife.

Sexual Pleasure for Both Partners

Islamic teachings tend to have a positive perspective towards sexual relationships. According to the Holy Qur'an, "*And of His signs is that He created for you from yourselves mates that you may find tranquility in them, and He placed between you affection and mercy*" (Q Ar-Rum 30:21). This is especially true regarding sexual satisfaction. Sex within marriage is described as a form of worship, where spouses are rewarded for satisfying each other sexually [7].

Islam does not restrict sex to reproduction, although it does describe it as an essential aspect of marriage. Both men and women have the right to sexual pleasure as a common spousal right. In cases where either spouse is unable to fulfil their sexual duties, divorce would be supported by the judge, and lack of satisfaction is grounds for annulment for both spouses. If a man suffers from impotence, all Muslim schools of thought agree that the woman has the right to an annulment or divorce [8].

Depriving one's spouse of their sexual rights is considered a sin. Women who deny their husbands their right to sex for reasons outside of sickness, tiredness, and menstruation could face legal repercussions, including loss of the right to financial alimony [9].

Masturbation

Although Islam highlights the right for sexual satisfaction between spouses, solitary pleasure outside of the context of marriage is discouraged. Most Islamic sects and schools of *fiqh* forbid masturbation to arouse oneself sexually. Most scholars believe that protecting one's genitals from sexual activities includes masturbation. According to the Holy Qur'an, "*Those who safeguard their chastity except from their spouses, or their dependents – then they are free from blame*" (Q Al-Mu'minun 23:5–6). However, when one has been unintentionally aroused, many scholars agree that masturbation in this case would be permissible, or *mubah*, to prevent *zina*, especially when the person is unmarried and is only practicing masturbation to control their sexual arousal rather than indulge in it, which applies the principle of "the lesser of two harms" that is widely applied within Islam. The rulings apply to men and women equally [10].

Male Circumcision and Female Genital Mutilation/Cutting

The rule within the Sunni school of thought is that circumcision is mandatory for boys [11]. Muslim communities and Muslim-majority countries have outlawed female genital mutilation/cutting (FGM/C). The recommendation of FGM/C is based on subjective interpretations and is often attributed to questionable or inauthentic Hadiths. There are neither clear definitive texts in the Qur'an nor authentic Hadith or Sunnah supporting FGM/C. On the contrary, apart from male circumcision, Islamic beliefs and principles strongly condemn any practice that negatively impacts the human body and "interferes with Allah's creation" in any way: "*And there is no changing Allah's creation. And that is the proper religion, but many people do not know*" (Q Ar-Rum 30:30) and "*make not your own hands contribute to your destruction*" (Q Al-Baqarah 2:195).

Views towards Contraception and Family Planning

The use of contraception is widely practiced and viewed as permissible in Islam as it is believed that God is merciful and would not intend for Muslims to suffer through having closely timed pregnancies or more children than they want. The Qur'an states: "*Allah desires for you ease; he desires no hardship for you*" (Q Al-Baqarah 2:185). Although contraception is generally acceptable among Muslim scholars for birth spacing, when practiced for birth limiting, it is a topic of continuous debate [12]. Withdrawal, or coitus interruptus, was widely practiced during the time of the Prophet Muhammad (PBUH) but required the wife's consent.

However, some scholars believe the use of surgical forms of contraception is forbidden irrespective of the purposes of use. All scholars agree that permanent methods (tubal ligation, hysterectomy, vasectomy) are forbidden in Islam and would only be allowed in cases of absolute necessity where there is a great danger to the mother's health and life [13]. Medical forms of contraception should be taken with close consideration to their effect on the woman's health as one of the main principles within Islamic jurisprudence is to prioritize nonmaleficence over beneficence.

Abortion

In the first 40 days of pregnancy, abortion is permitted by most Muslim schools of thought, and the decision is mutual between spouses. Other scholars permitted abortion up to 120 days from conception when the "soul develops." However, specific circumstances need to be met to allow abortion within this timeframe. These include, but are not limited to, fetal deformity, rape, incest, and physical or mental inability to raise children [14]. After 120 days, abortion would only be allowed in the case of fetal death and in cases where terminating a pregnancy is crucial to save a mother's life [14]. However, two requirements must be met first to allow abortion after the 120-day point. Firstly, a panel of two or three specialist doctors (depending on the local regulations of the country) and the hospital director must sign and agree that the continuation of the pregnancy would lead to the mother's death, or that all measures to save the fetus have been exhausted. The second requirement is the permission of her husband [14].

Islamic Views regarding Assisted Reproduction

The treatment of infertility is permitted in Islam for married couples. Assisted reproductive technology refers to any medical procedure used to address infertility including in vitro fertilization (IVF) and intrauterine insemination (IUI). Assisted reproduction is permissible in Islam under the following strict conditions. First, the sperm and ovum must come from legally married couples. Second, the embryo should be implanted in the uterus of the wife. Third, the procedure must be done during the span of their marriage. Furthermore, all measures should be taken to eliminate the risk of mixing sperm, eggs, or zygotes of different couples [15]. Concerns over the possibility of mixing frozen embryos were raised by some Islamic scholars; therefore, all measures should be taken to ensure that embryos are the exclusive property of the couple and are not to be transferred to others [15]. It is also permissible to freeze the remaining embryos to be used by the same couple in subsequent IVF cycles within their marriage period [15].

Third-Party Assistance: Egg and Sperm Donation and Surrogacy

The involvement of a third party in the reproductive process between a married couple is forbidden under Islamic law [16]. This includes the use of a third-party sperm, ovum, embryo, or uterus. As such, egg and sperm donation and surrogacy are prohibited in Islam [15]. The Islamic Fiqh Council allowed surrogacy between the wives of the same husband in 1984. This *fatwa* was withdrawn in 1985 [16]. The opposition to surrogacy is based on the assumption that a woman is carrying a fertilized egg of a man who is not her husband, which is therefore considered a form of *zina* [17].

Oocyte Cryopreservation

Oocyte cryopreservation, also known as egg freezing, is a medical procedure done to preserve a woman's eggs. This procedure is used to enable women to postpone pregnancy for medical or social reasons. Egg freezing for medical reasons is permissible in Islam [15]. Examples of medical reasons include treatments that could impact egg production, such as radiation and chemotherapy. However, egg freezing for social reasons is debatable in Islam. Some Islamic scholars disapprove of the procedure for single women to delay marriage. Another reason is the fear of mixing frozen eggs, thereby tainting ancestry [18]. However, a *fatwa* issued in 2019 permitted egg freezing for single women subject to specific conditions [19]. For example, the egg must be used by the same woman, it should be fertilized by the future husband within the timeframe of a valid marriage, and the egg must be stored safely to prevent possible mixing.

Sex Selection

Sex selection for medical reasons is permitted to prevent illness (e.g., sex-linked illnesses) [15]. However, sex selection for social reasons is controversial as Muslims scholars feared its use to discriminate against females [15]. Therefore, it was permitted for social reasons when the following conditions were met [20]. First, sex selection should not be used for the first child. Second, it should not be used to ensure only one sex in all children in the family. Third, the use of sex selection technologies to have children from both sexes in the family will preserve the mother's health if she has had multiple pregnancies, difficult pregnancies, or high-risk pregnancies [16].

Medication to Induce Ovulation

Ovulatory stimulants, such as clomiphene, are used to induce egg production. The use of medication to induce ovulation is permissible in Islam for treating infertility. It is also permissible to use for couples who wish to have twins. The use of ovulatory stimulants is permissible under the condition that a competent doctor is consulted before its use to ensure no harm is caused to the mother [21].

Sexual and Reproductive Health Services in Islam

Sex and Religious Background of Health Care Professionals

According to Islamic bioethics, a suggestive hierarchy of physicians to attend to Muslim patients is as follows: a Muslim physician of the same sex, a non-Muslim physician of the same sex, a Muslim physician of the opposite sex, and, finally, a non-Muslim physician of the opposite sex [22]. The prioritization of the sex of health care professionals stems from the high value of preventing *khalwah* (a state in which a male is alone with a woman other than his wife or a woman to whom by reason of consanguinity, affinity, or fosterage he is forbidden by Muslim Law to marry) and preserving *awrah* (the intimate parts of the human body that must be covered under Islamic law), which is more tolerable in same-sex interactions [22]. The preference for health care professionals from the same religion stems from the belief that Muslim health care providers would be able to support Muslim patients with medical treatments while preserving religious rulings. Regardless of this suggestive hierarchy, Islamic ruling allows for situations where deviation from the rule is allowed. In case of medical emergency and based on the principle of "necessity makes for allowing the prohibited," Muslims can receive care from any competent health care professional regardless of their sex or religious background [22].

The Presence of a Companion during the Medical Examination

The presence of a companion during a medical consultation is required to address the prohibition of *khalwah* between patients and health care providers of the opposite sex. Ideally, a companion of the same sex as the patient should be close enough to the patient to be able to hear the consultation and to disrupt seclusion [22]. This is consistent with a universal practice that necessitates the presence of chaperones when conducting sensitive medical examinations by a physician from the opposite sex.

Husband's Consent for Medical Procedures

A husband's consent to the wife's medical procedures is not required within Islamic law. In cases of the medical necessity of reproductive medical procedures, such as a hysterectomy, an oophorectomy, or a cesarean section, the woman should give consent and authorize the procedure herself [23]. A male guardian's consent on medically necessary procedures is not required as a competent woman is more knowledgeable of her interests. However, within many Muslim-majority countries, patriarchal rules continue to limit women's autonomy by demanding the husband's approval for various medical and surgical procedures [24].

Conclusion

Sex within Islam is not restricted to procreation; rather, the right to pleasure is ensured for both men and women if it is practiced within the institution of marriage. In fact, marriage can be dissolved in the case of impotence or refusal to sexually satisfy the spouse. However, different views exist on masturbation, which can be permissible in specific situations and prohibited in others. Family planning, both natural and medical, is permissible by most Muslim scholars when mutually agreed upon by both spouses and used for spacing children rather than limiting them. Fertility treatments are also permissible if the marriage is active and only the current spouses are involved in the treatment. Modern reproductive issues like oocyte cryotherapy are subjected to different Islamic scholarly opinions, but they mostly lean to permissibility, unlike surrogacy which is mostly prohibited by most Muslim scholars. Accessing sexual health services is allowed and encouraged in Islam. Although there is encouragement for each sex to seek medical advice from professionals of the same sex, preserving one's life and health is always prioritized over any restrictions. Women do not need to seek their husband's approval for medical procedures aimed at saving life, yet in many Muslim-majority countries restrictions to women's autonomy regarding medical consent exist.

References

1. Islam, M. Z. Interfaith marriage in Islam and present situation. *Global Journal of Politics and Law Research*. 2014;2(1):36–47.

2. Khadduri, M. Marriage in Islamic law: the modernist viewpoints. *The American Journal of Comparative Law*. 1978;26(2):213–18. https://doi.org/10.2307/839669

3. Leeman, A. B. Interfaith marriage in Islam: an examination of the legal theory behind the traditional and reformist positions. *Indiana Law Journal*. 2009;84:743.

4. Bello, A. H. The punishment for adultery in Islamic law and its application in Nigeria. *Journal of Islamic Law and Culture*. 2011;13(2–3):166–82. https://doi.org/10.1080/1528817X.2012.733132

5. Rasool, S. & Suleman, M. Muslim women overcoming marital violence: breaking through "structural and cultural prisons" created by religious leaders. *Agenda*. 2016;30(3):39–49. https://doi.org/10.1080/10130950.2016.1275199

6. Mashhour, A. Islamic law and gender equality: could there be a common ground? A study of divorce and polygamy in Sharia Law and contemporary legislation in Tunisia and Egypt. *Human Rights Quarterly*. 2005;27(2):562–96. http://dx.doi.org/10.1353/hrq.2005.0022

7. an-Nawawi. *Hadith 25, 40 Hadith an-Nawawi*. Available from: https://sunnah.com/nawawi40:25

8. Jawad Mughniyya, M. Marriage according to the Five Schools of Islamic Law: Al-'Anan (impotence). [online]. n.d. [Accessed January 3, 2023]. Available from: www.al-islam.org/marriage-according-five-schools-islamic-law-muhammad-jawad-mughniyya/al-uyub-defects

9. Alsaggaf, A. A. The definition of disobedience. [online]. 2022 [Accessed January 4, 2023]. Available from: https://dorar.net/feqhia/5335/

10. Islamqa. Alaistimna' eind khashyat alzina [Masturbation for fear of fornication]. [online]. 2020 [Accessed January 3, 2023]. Available from: https://islamqa.info/ar/answers/317498/

11. The Permanent Committee for Scholarly Research. Ruling on circumcision: Part No. 4; Page No. 423. [online]. 2022 [Accessed March 3, 2023]. Available from: https://alifta.gov.sa/

12. Roudi-Fahimi, F. *Islam and Family Planning*. Population Reference Bureau. 2004. Available from: www.prb.org/wp-content/uploads/2004/09/IslamFamilyPlanning.pdf

13. The Permanent Committee for Scholarly Research. Decision of the Council of Senior Scholars regarding birth control: Part No. 19, Page No. 297. [online]. 2022 [Accessed March 3, 2023]. Available from: https://alifta.gov.sa/

14. Hessini, L. Abortion and Islam: policies and practice in the Middle East and North Africa. *Reproductive Health Matters*. 2007;15(29):75–84. https://doi.org/10.1016/s0968-8080(06)29279-6

15. Al-Bar, M. A. & Chamsi-Pasha, H. Assisted reproductive technology: Islamic perspective. In: Mohammed Ali Al-Bar & Hassan Chamsi-Pasha, eds. *Contemporary Bioethics: Islamic perspective*. New York: Springer. 2015. 173–86.

16. Khan, M. A. & Konje, J. C. Ethical and religious dilemmas of modern reproductive choices and the Islamic perspective. *European Journal of Obstetrics & Gynecology and Reproductive Biology*. 2019;232:5–9. https://doi.org/10.1016/j.ejogrb.2018.10.052

17. Deonandan, R. Thoughts on the ethics of gestational surrogacy: perspectives from religions, Western liberalism, and comparisons with adoption. *Journal of Assisted Reproduction and Genetics*. 2020;37(2):269–79. https://doi.org/10.1007/s10815-019-01647-y

18. Chin, A. H. B. & Saifuddeen, S. M. Is social egg freezing (oocyte cryopreservation) for single women permissible in Islam? A perspective from Singapore. *The New Bioethics*. 2022;28(2):1–11. https://doi.org/10.1080/20502877.2022.2063576

19. Alawi, S. Egg freezing permissible in Islam, according to Egypt's Dar Al-Ifta. [online]. Harvard Law. 2019 [Accessed January 8, 2023]. Available from: https://blog.petrieflom.law.harvard.edu/2019/09/23/egg-freezing-permissible-in-islam-according-to-egypts-dar-al-ifta/

20. Serour, G. I. Islamic perspectives in human reproduction. *Reproductive Biomedicine Online*. 2008;17:34–38. https://doi.org/10.1016/s1472-6483(10)60328-8

21. Islamqa. Hukm 'akhdh munashitat lihamil bitawayim [Ruling on taking stimulants to conceive twins]. 2009 [Accessed March 3, 2023]. Available from: https://islamqa.info/ar/answers/134502/

22. Padela, A. I. & del Pozo, P. R. Muslim patients and cross-gender interactions in medicine: an Islamic bioethical

perspective. *Journal of Medical Ethics.* 2011;37(1):40–44. https://doi.org/10 .1136/jme.2010.037614

23. Resolution CoSS. Bishan alhusul ealaa muafaqat alzawjayn ealaa eamaliaat aistisal alrahim walmabyad waleamaliaat alqaysaria [No. 173: on the obtainment of both spouses' consent in hysterectomies, oophorectomies, and cesarean sections].

1992 [Accessed February 4, 2023]. Available from: https://alifta.net/

24. Alomair, N., Alageel, S., Davies, N., & Bailey, J. V. Factors influencing sexual and reproductive health of Muslim women: a systematic review. *Reproductive Health.* 2020;17(1):1–15. https://doi.org/ 10.1186/s12978-020-0888-1

Zakat and Waqf: Towards Achieving Sustainability, Health, and Well-Being

Mohammad Abdullah

Introduction

Charity is quintessential of Islamic rewardable activities. From among the various forms of Sharia-prescribed charities, zakat and waqf emerged as the leading redistributive tools, and these two assumed institutional shapes. The Sharia prescription of zakat originates from the Qur'an, whereas the conceptual premises of waqf are derived from the Prophetic traditions [1]. Zakat is obligatory once a year for Muslims who meet the Sharia-prescribed criteria and threshold. The heads of zakat beneficiaries are well-defined in the primary sources of Sharia [2]. In comparison, waqf implies a voluntary form of charity that can be exercised by anyone who could afford to do so at any moment [3]. There is no Sharia restriction on who can make a waqf or who can benefit from it so far as the process and purpose of its exercise and the usage do not conflict with the fundamentals of Sharia [4]. Both zakat and waqf have a history of contribution to the socioeconomic development of Muslim communities [5].

The repeated Sharia prescription and encouragement of charity in the Qur'an imply its vision of inculcating altruistic behavior in Muslims, which helps to develop a mutually supportive, cohesive, and inclusive society [6]. The institutional philosophy of Islamic charitable institutions may be construed in light of the critical role of custodianship that the human being has been assigned by Allah. As such, the Islamic belief system envisages the role of human beings as the custodian of the planet Earth. To remain true to this responsibility, human beings are commanded to ensure the survival of fellow human beings through various means and modes of charity [1].

From an Islamic perspective, the issue of health and well being is crucial. Sharia lays great emphasis on ensuring the health and well-being of all. From the prism of *Maqasid al-Shariah* (the higher objectives of Sharia), striving to maintain a healthy lifestyle and enabling others to achieve health and well-being are among the desired objectives. Importantly, the objective of health and well-being is included in the UN-endorsed program of sustainable development – which is encapsulated in the Sustainable Development Goals (SDGs) – as part of the first three goals. This is broadly in affinity with the Sharia paradigm of sustainability and sustainable development [7].

This chapter delves into the modern relevance of two critical Islamic charitable institutions, zakat and waqf, followed by examining their importance, particularly in the context of health and well-being.

Sharia, Sustainability, and the Role of Islamic Charitable Institutions

Sharia constitutes a set of divine principles, beliefs, and ethical norms. Its construct is founded on the instructions received from Allah, the Lawgiver. It guides mankind in different spheres of their lives through its prescribed principles, values, and rules [8], which are found in the Qur'an and Sunnah, its primary sources. Within the prism of Sharia, humans have been delegated the responsibility of custodianship to this Earth. Thus, the care and affairs of this planet have been handed over to human beings in the capacity of a trustee or deputy. This understanding is based on the Qur'anic verse in which the Creator Himself explains the projected role of human beings at the very inception. The Qur'an says, "*(Remember) when your Lord said to the angels, I am going to create a deputy on the earth!*" (Q Al-Baqarah 2:30).

As part of this responsibility, it is envisioned that the human – as the trustee/custodian of this planet – remains conscious of their actions and activities and adopt responsible behavior. To play the role of trustee, humans need to be considerate to the habitants of planet Earth and help them maintain a sustainable lifestyle. Among the key constituents of such an approach include avoidance of extravagance, extreme actions, irresponsible patterns of production, and consumption. Rather, a balanced, moderate, and diligent approach towards nature and its habitants is warranted.

The role of Islamic charitable institutions in supporting people and the planet is critical [9]. Charities provide an instrumental support system to society by supplying necessities and creating sustainable safety nets for deserving people and righteous purposes [10]. To be aligned with the *Maqasid al-Shariah*, charities are required to be conducted through environment-friendly modes and schemes. In fact, the *Maqasid*-based exercise of charity is vital for the survival of people and the planet.

Waqf and Its Role in Supporting Health and Well-Being

Charity forms an indispensable part of Islamic religious activities. Numerous verses of the Qur'an lay great emphasis on charity and charitable activities while encouraging righteous and rewardable deeds. For example, in Q Al-Baqarah 2:43, the Qur'an says, "*Be steadfast in prayer; practice regular charity and bow down with those who bow down (in worship).*" Similarly, in Q Al-Hadeed 57:18, the Qur'an states, "*For those who give in charity, men, and women, and loan to Allah a beautiful loan, it shall be increased manifold.*" There are multiple forms of charity outlined within the Qur'an and Hadith, the primary sources of Sharia. Charity in these sources is mainly categorized into obligatory and voluntary types [11]. While zakat and *Sadaqah al-fitr* fall under the obligatory forms of charity, a general *Sadaqah* constitutes voluntary charity. In Sharia, an obligatory form of charity has a relatively restrictive set of rules and parameters. Comparatively, a voluntary charity is flexible. The institution of waqf constitutes a voluntary form of charity. Notwithstanding its voluntary nature, waqf has been instrumental in spearheading charitable activities and dispensation of wealth to the needy and deserving throughout Islamic history [12].

Waqf refers to a distinct form of Islamic philanthropic institution. The distinction of waqf over other forms of Islamic charities is demarcated by its principal condition of sustainability. Theoretically, the inspiration for waqf is believed to have originated from those Qur'anic verses which exhort charity, almsgiving, and voluntary disposition of wealth for the sake of Allah. In the literature of Islamic jurisprudence, the terms waqf and *habs* were coined by jurists and frequently employed to capture the essence of what is referred to in the Hadith as *Sadaqah jariyah* [13].

In view of its special spiritual merit and critical socioeconomic function, waqf rapidly became a well-familiarized institution among Muslim societies and successfully secured a distinctive place across Muslim regions. In a historical context, waqf is attributed to have made an enormous contribution towards the establishment of Islamic civilization. Among the list of critical contributions of waqf include the development of hospitals, medical research centers, health care facilities, public infrastructure, wells, canals, inns, parks, roads, free drinking water, and food arrangements. Historically, poor, pauper, and underprivileged people have been the greatest beneficiaries of waqf [14].

By virtue of its flexible nature and jurisprudence, the institution of waqf has been dynamic in accommodating the newly arising needs of different societies. The institution of waqf equally provided for the wealthy as much as it supported the deprived and have-nots in Muslim society. Compared to other forms of Islamic charities, waqf gained wider acceptability and recognition among Muslim societies, perhaps due to the flexibility this institution offers in encompassing a myriad of social causes, purposes, and objectives [15]. The nature of dynamism in waqf may be gauged by the fact that a waqf is fit to serve any objectives of social needs so far as an objective is not in contradiction with the fundamentals of Sharia [16].

Given its built-in flexibility and massive institutional capacity, it is envisaged that waqf stands out in supporting sustainable development by supplying charitable resources at a marginal cost. For this, as postulated by some recent literature, the role of waqf may be contextualized by juxtaposing the objectives that this institution has historically served with the SDGs in general and, in particular, the third SDG on achieving health and well-being for all. It is argued that most of SDGs are in affinity with the objectives of Sharia and, thus, may be prioritized by waqf, particularly across the Muslim nations [7]. Waqf may play a crucial role in targeting the third SDG by providing the critical resources required for ensuring the health and well-being of all [17]. It is estimated that the value of total waqfs globally exceeds one trillion dollars [7]. Considering its mammoth size and scale, global waqfs may be a change agent in providing the pitch for sustainable development.

Zakat and Its Role in Sustainable Development

Though the concept and application of charity is often linked with volunteerism and thus is treated as an optional activity in a religious context, Sharia prescribes both forms of charity: voluntary and obligatory [18]. Zakat in Sharia is a mandatory form of charity that constitutes one of the five key pillars of Islam. The primary sources of Sharia not only enjoin the believers to perform zakat as a mandatory form of charity but also term it as one of the signs of true believers in Allah and Hereafter. The Qur'an states, "*Who believe in the unseen, establish prayer, and donate from what We have provided for them*" (Q Al-Baqarah 2:3). Compared to salat, which is compulsory for all Muslims five times a day, the obligation of zakat occurs once in a year and is limited to the qualifiers of zakat-related specific criteria.

Zakat forms one of the five essentials of Islam and is mentioned more than 80 times in the Qur'an. In the context of financial worship, zakat finds repeated references in prophetic traditions as well [2]. Based on zakat jurisprudence, it is an agreed-upon rule that zakat applies only to certain types of wealth and is obligatory upon specific categories of people meeting the zakat-specific criteria [2]. In addition, this financial worship of Islam is to be performed only once a year and is meant to support specific heads of beneficiaries. Thus, there is less flexibility in terms of who can perform zakat and who can benefit from it, as both aspects are strictly defined in the primary sources of Sharia.

Among the key requirements of zakat obligation includes the primary criterion that a specific wealth shall be Sharia-recognized and zakat-able (i.e., eligible for zakat). Similarly, the wealth shall reach the minimum threshold of zakat and shall be owned by a specific individual for at least one year. There are different minimum thresholds of zakat for different categories of zakat-able assets. Principally, the threshold of zakat is defined in gold and silver. The defined threshold of zakat in the primary sources of Sharia for gold and silver is generally converted as 85 grams of gold and 595 grams of silver. The minimum threshold of either of these two metals should be owned by a specific individual for a lunar year of 354 days. The applicable rate of zakat is 2.5% of zakat-able items which is calculated on the passage of a complete lunar year on the ownership of wealth [2].

There are eight clearly determined heads that can be offered zakat benefits. In this context, zakat is relatively a nonflexible institution compared to waqf and other forms of optional charities. The heads of zakat beneficiaries are elaborated in the Qur'anic verse Q At-Tawbah 9:60, which states, "*Alms are only for the poor and the needy, for those employed to collect it and to attract the hearts of those who have been inclined (towards Islam), and to free the captives, and for those in debt, and for Allah's way, and the wayfarer; a duty imposed by Allah.*"

Zakat has positive effects on encouraging investment tendency, reducing the fiscal burden of governments for supporting charitable and social causes, accelerating economic activities, and creating a harmonious environment. Zakat also plays a critical role in reducing the gap between the rich and poor in providing for the poor and underprivileged [19]. The objectives of zakat include both materials as well as spiritual benefits for the zakat payer. Cleansing the heart and mind from the much-abhorred trait of greed and voracity for mundane belongings is one of the spiritual objectives of zakat obligation. Also, the purification of wealth from which zakat is due is another spiritual objective. The Qur'an states, "*Take alms of their wealth, wherewith thou mayst purify them and mayst make them grow, and pray for them. Lo! thy prayer is an assuagement for them. Allah is Hearer, Knower*" (Q At-Tawbah 9:103).

Sustainability, Sustainable Development, and Islamic Charities

The role of charity is critical in reducing imbalance in society that causes disharmony among different categories of people. Also, the role of charity is pivotal in safeguarding the masses from various forms of deprivation. It is also critical in uplifting the poor from the burden of extreme poverty. The significance of charity increases in scenarios where there is either a deficiency of public goods or a scarcity of sufficient funds to be distributed among the poor in the form of basic allowance. Zakat and waqf, being the primary two charitable institutions of Sharia, are meant to care for the poor and underprivileged on an ongoing basis. Most of the required resources for a society can be supplied by the institutions of waqf and zakat in a sustainable manner [19].

In the context of sustainable development, it is argued that most of the SDGs are amenable to Sharia's objectives. There are several interlinkages between SDGs and Islamic charitable institutions [7]. Waqf and zakat have historically provided resources to Muslim societies to achieve and maintain health and well-being on a sustainable basis. These two institutions have been critical in alleviating poverty, ending hunger, and providing the means for health and well-being. The institution of waqf has a track record of supplying necessities and helping the smooth functioning of society. Being an obligatory form of charity, zakat on the other hand provides a more predictable and certain source of funds for socioeconomic purposes. If deployed strategically and sustainably, the two institutions may play an instrumental role in helping Muslim-majority nations achieve sustainable development.

Conclusion

In Sharia, the objective of charity is two-dimensional: to encourage the redistribution of wealth from the wealthy to the poor, and to ensure the purification of wealth. The first objective is envisaged to help create an environment of cooperation among fellow beings, and the second is meant to entail a spiritually healthy state of heart and mind for the donor. This chapter delineated the concept, mechanism, and operational frameworks of zakat (Islamic obligatory charity) and waqf (Islamic endowment) and discussed their potential roles in achieving the third SDG in particular. The chapter argued that there is an inherent consistency between the higher objectives of Sharia and the sustainable development agenda of the world community.

Charity forms an integral constituent of Islamic societies. The institutions of waqf and zakat are at the forefront of the third sector of an Islamic economy. Although the nature of these two institutions is different from an obligatory and nonobligatory perspective, their roles in supporting the people and planet have been of almost equal merit. While zakat is a mandatory form of charity and is performed once a year, waqf is an optional charity and can be exercised at any time.

To highlight their positive roles, the resources of these two institutions need to be applied in tandem with *Maqasid al-Shariah*. The *Maqasid*-based developmental approach entails accommodating the essentials of sustainability. A responsible approach towards the utilization of Islamic charitable resources is crucial for optimizing their roles and contribution. In addition, the benefits of Islamic charities can be effectively cascaded to future generations only if their usage is aligned with the requisites of *Maqasid al-Shariah*. Thus, by integrating the objectives of Sharia into zakat and waqf distribution and application policies, the utility of their resources can be improved and the reach of their benefits can be expanded. This may ultimately result in developing a sustainable, progressive, and smooth-functioning society.

References

1. Abdullah, M. Religion and development: an Islamic approach to socio-economic development. In: Burki, U. Azid, T, & Dahlstrom, R., eds. *Foundations of a* *Sustainable Economy*. Abingdon, UK: Routledge. 2021. 121–38.

2. Al-Qardawi, Y. Kahf, M., trans. *Fiqh al-Zakat*. London: Dar al-Taqwa Ltd. 1985.

3. Abdullah, M. Waqf, social responsibility, and real economy. In: Saiti, B. & Sarea, A., eds. *Challenges and Impacts of Religious Endowments on Global Economics and Finance.* Hershey, PA: IGI Global. 2020. 23–36.

4. Abdullah, M. Waqf and trust: the nature, structures and socio-economic impacts. *Journal of Islamic Accounting and Business Research.* 2019;10:512–27. https://doi.org/10.1108/JIABR-10-2016-0124

5. Lev, Y. *Charity, Endowments and Charitable Institutions in Medieval Islam.* Gainesville, FL: University Press of Florida. 2005.

6. Abdullah, M. Analysing the moral aspect of qard: a Shariah perspective. *International Journal of Islamic and Middle Eastern Finance and Management.* 2015;8:171–84. https://doi.org/10.1108/IMEFM-11-2013-0116

7. Abdullah, M. Waqf, Sustainable Development Goals (SDGs) and maqasid al-shariah. *International Journal of Social Economics.* 2018;45:158–72. https://doi.org/10.1108/IJSE-10-2016-0295

8. Kamali, H. M. *Maqasid al-Shariah, Ijtihad and Civilisational Renewal.* London: The International Institute of Islamic Thought. 2012.

9. Çizakça, M. *A History of Philanthropic Foundations: The Islamic World from the Seventh Century to the Present.* Istanbul: Bogazici University Press. 2000.

10. Ahmad, H., Mohieldin, M., Verbeek, J., & Aboulmagd, F. *On the Sustainable Development Goals and the Role of Islamic Finance.* Washington, DC: World Bank Group. 2015.

11. Abdullah, M. Objectives of awqaf within the classical discourse and their modern implications. In: Billah M., ed. *Awqaf-led Islamic Social Finance.* Abingdon, UK: Routledge. 2020. 23–38.

12. Sabra, A. *Poverty and Charity in Medieval Islam: Mumluk Egypt. 1250–1517.* Cambridge: Cambridge University Press. 2000.

13. Abdullah, M. Classical waqf, juristic analogy and framework of awqaf doctrines. *ISRA International Journal of Islamic Finance.* 2020;12(2):281–96. https://doi.org/10.1108/IJIF-07-2019-0102

14. Abdullah, M. Islamic endowment (waqf) in India: towards poverty reduction of Muslims in the country. *Journal of Research in Emerging Markets.* 2020;2(2):48–60.

15. Abdullah, M. Evolution in waqf jurisprudence and Islamic financial innovation. *Journal of Islamic Monetary Economics and Finance.* 2018;4:161–82. https://doi.org/10.21098/jimf.v4i1.920

16. Abdullah, M. A new framework of corporate governance of waqf: a preliminary proposal. *Islam and Civilisational Renewal.* 2015;6(3):353–70.

17. Securities Commission Malaysia. *Harnessing Waqf into a Bankable Social Financing and Investment Asset Class.* Proceedings of the SC-OCIS Roundtable 2014. Kuala Lumpur: SC-OCIS. 2015.

18. Singer, A. *Charity in Islamic Societies.* Cambridge: Cambridge University Press. 2008.

19. Ben Jedidia, K. & Guerbouj, K. Effects of zakat on the economic growth in selected Islamic countries: empirical evidence. *International Journal of Development Issues.* 2021;20:126–42. https://doi.org/10.1108/IJDI-05-2020-0100

Earth and the Environment: Islam and Stewardship

Khaled Obaideen, Ied Shukur Alnidawi

Introduction

Religious teachings play a significant role in human behavior, ethical frameworks, and perceptions of the world across various historical periods. Islam, one of the world's major religions, guides spirituality, human relations, and environmental protection. The environment and its diverse components, ranging from expansive bodies of water to the smallest of insects, are frequently cited in Islamic teachings [1]. The references to natural elements are not limited to mere backdrops or metaphors but are regarded as integral elements of the intricate tapestry of existence that God (Allah) has designed. Islam emphasizes the importance of nature and the ethical obligation of humans to act as stewards, as evident in its foundational texts, namely the Holy Qur'an and the Prophetic Hadith, which consist of the teachings and actions of Prophet Muhammad (PBUH).

Due to escalating global environmental crises, such as climate change, water scarcity, and biodiversity loss, there is an increasing imperative to comprehend the intrinsic environmental values inherent in Islamic traditions [2]. This chapter explores the comprehensive viewpoint of Islam regarding environmental stewardship, providing valuable insights into how Islamic teachings can offer culturally congruent guidance in addressing present-day environmental challenges.

Islamic Creation Story and Human's Role

The Holy Qur'an, Islam's holy book, describes the creation of the Earth and the universe: *"He it is Who created for you all that is on Earth. Then He rose over towards the heaven and made them seven heavens and He is the All-Knower of everything"* (Q Al-Baqarah 2:29). This verse underscores the deliberate and intricate design of the Earth, tailored to cater to human needs and all other forms of life.

Central to the creation narrative is the story of Adam (PBUH), the first human according to Islamic scripture. While other creatures were made to inhabit the Earth, Adam held a unique position. Allah says, *"And when your Lord said to the angels, 'Indeed, I will make upon the earth a successive authority (Khalifah).' They said, 'Will You place upon it one who causes corruption therein and sheds blood, while we declare Your praise and sanctify You?' He [Allah] said, 'Indeed, I know that which you do not know.'"* (Q Al-Baqarah 2:30). The term *Khalifah* or "steward" implies that humans, beginning with Adam, are endowed with both authority and responsibility. They are entrusted to take care of the Earth and not exploit it.

Furthermore, Adam was bestowed with knowledge, which distinguished him from other creatures: *"And He taught Adam the names – all of them. Then He showed them to the angels and said, 'Inform Me of the names of these, if you are truthful.'"* (Q Al-Baqarah 2:31). This knowledge comes with the responsibility to use it judiciously, respecting the limits set by Allah.

Qur'anic Verses Related to Nature

The Holy Qur'an contains many verses highlighting the beauty, complexity, and significance of nature, often using it as a means to reflect on the greatness of Allah [3]. Nature, in the Qur'anic perspective, is not a passive backdrop but an active testament to God's power, wisdom, and mercy.

Important verses discussing nature and the environment include the following:

1. Creation and Balance: *"It is He who spread out the earth and placed therein firmly set mountains and rivers; and of all the fruits He placed therein two spouses. He covers the night with the day. Indeed in that are signs (Ayat) for people who reflect"* (Q Ar-Ra'd 13:3). This verse reflects on the meticulous design and balance in creation.
2. Water as a Source of Life: *"And We have made from water every living thing. Then will they not believe?"* (Q Al-Anbiya 21:30). Here, water's fundamental role in creating and sustaining life is emphasized.
3. Mountains as Stabilizers: *"Have We not made the earth a resting place? And the mountains as stakes?"* (Q An-Naba' 78:6–7). Mountains are described as pegs, suggesting their role in stabilizing the Earth.
4. The Interconnectedness of Life: *"And there is no creature on [or within] the earth or bird that flies with its wings except [that they are] communities like you. We have not neglected in the Register a thing. Then unto their Lord, they will be gathered"* (Q Al-An'am 6:38). This underscores the idea that every creature has a purpose and role in the ecosystem.

One of the recurring themes in the Holy Qur'an is the portrayal of nature. These themes include:

1. A Reminder of God's Existence and Attribute: *"Indeed, in the creation of the heavens and the earth and the alternation of the night and the day are signs for those of understanding"* (Q Al 'Imran 3:190).
2. Reflection and Contemplation: Nature serves as a means for humans to reflect upon, leading to a deeper understanding of themselves and their Creator.
3. Gratitude: observing the benefits and blessings inherent in nature, humans are reminded to be grateful to God.
4. Moral and Ethical Lessons: Nature often serves as a parable, illustrating moral and spiritual truths.

Muslims are instructed to study and contemplate nature in the Holy Qur'an. This ideology fosters a sense of reverence for the natural world and emphasizes the ethical obligation to safeguard and maintain it.

Prophetic Hadiths Concerning the Environment

The Prophetic Hadith serves as a supplement to the Holy Qur'an, guiding various topics, including the area of environmental ethics. The Prophetic Hadiths not only offer practical guidelines but also emphasize the fundamental moral principles that form the basis of Islamic teachings regarding nature and the environment [4]:

1. Conservation of Resources: The Prophet Muhammad (PBUH) said, "Do not waste water, even if you perform your ablution on the banks of an abundantly flowing river" [5]. This Hadith underscores the principle of conservation and the responsible use of even abundant resources.

2. Planting Trees and Greenery: The Prophet Muhammad (PBUH) stated, "If a Muslim plants a tree or sows seeds, and then a bird, or a person, or an animal eats from it, it is regarded as a charitable gift (Sadaqah) for him" [6]. This Hadith emphasizes the virtues of planting trees and the broader concept of sustainable and beneficial actions for the environment.

3. Treatment of Animals: Prophet Muhammad (PBUH) narrated, "Whoever kills a bird or anything bigger than that without a just cause, Allah will hold him accountable on the Day of Judgment" [7]. This saying emphasizes the ethical treatment of all creatures, regardless of their size.

4. Avoiding Harm to the Environment: Prophet Muhammad (PBUH) stated, "Beware of the three acts that cause you to be cursed: relieving yourselves in shaded places (that people utilize), in a walkway or in a watering place" [8]. This Hadith underscores the importance of maintaining cleanliness and not causing harm to communal spaces.

5. Waste and Excess: The Prophet Muhammad (PBUH) advised, "The worst vessel to fill is the stomach. Enough for the son of Adam is a few morsels to keep his back straight. But if he must, then one-third for food, one-third for drink, and one-third for air" [9]. This Hadith promotes moderation in consumption and warns against wastefulness.

The Hadiths serve to reinforce the emphasis found in the Qur'an regarding the importance of environmental stewardship. They guide believers on how to coexist harmoniously with the natural world while also highlighting the moral and ethical responsibilities towards all aspects of creation.

Principles of Environmental Ethics in Islam

The environmental ethics of Islam are rooted in various fundamental principles that are present in both the Holy Qur'an and Prophetic Hadith. These principles serve as a guiding framework for Muslims in their interactions with the natural world [10].

The fundamental principle of Islam is the concept of Tawhid, which refers to the belief in the Oneness of God [11]. This statement underscores the notion that every creation serves as a manifestation of God's indivisibility, sagacity, and deliberate arrangement. This perspective also emphasizes two primary concepts: a) the inherent interconnectedness within the natural world, emphasizing that any damage inflicted upon a specific component of the ecosystem has repercussions on the entirety, and b) the belief that natural phenomena serve as symbolic indications or ayat, providing individuals with a profound understanding and connection to the Divine Creator.

The principle of Khalifah, which emphasizes stewardship, posits that humans are entrusted with the responsibility of caring for the Earth rather than asserting ownership over it. The role of guardianship not only entails the protection of the environment but also promotes the sense of responsibility that Muslims bear. Muslims hold the belief that their behaviors, encompassing their interactions with the environment, will undergo divine examination in the celestial realm beyond mortal existence.

The emphasis placed on balance (*Mizan*) in the Holy Qur'an signifies the presence of harmony within the natural world [11]. All natural phenomena, ranging from the cyclical changes of seasons to the complex interplay of ecosystems, function within a clearly defined and harmonious system. Disruptions to this equilibrium, such as excessive consumption or environmental contamination, conflict with the sacred design. Islam also advocates for moderation in human actions, emphasizing the importance of avoiding excessive behavior.

The principle of wastefulness, known as *Israf*, is emphasized in Islam [12]. The act of both utilizing and wasting resources is generally disapproved of. The Prophet Muhammad (PBUH) provided explicit guidance discouraging the inappropriate utilization of vital resources, such as water. The concept of wastefulness encompasses both material and spiritual dimensions, the latter of which supports the notion that indulgence and extravagance signify a lack of appreciation for the blessings bestowed by the Divine, potentially resulting in hubris and disconnection from divine guidance.

Islamic Environmental Practices

Islam blends philosophy and practice, especially in environmental issues. The faith's high-level principles also provide practical guidelines for daily life, ensuring believers live in harmony with nature [13].

Water, symbolizing both life and purity, is central to Islamic rituals. *Wudu*, or ablution, before prayers emphasizes cleanliness. Purification and conservation are considered priorities. The Prophet Muhammad (PBUH) often performed *wudu* with little water. His advice against wasting water, even by a fast-flowing river, emphasizes conservation and gratitude, reminding believers not to take abundant resources for granted. This conservationist approach includes resource consumption. Believers should consume mindfully and avoid waste to thank Allah for His blessings [14].

Islamic teachings also mention forests, trees, and the importance of environmental ecology [4]. Planting trees is considered a charitable act with rewards for helping animals [2]. Even during the war, the Prophet Muhammad (PBUH) promoted tree protection and discouraged their felling, emphasizing their value.

Islam's compassion extends to caring for and protecting animals. Like humans, animals have rights according to the faith. They should be cared for and not overworked [15]. Numerous anecdotes from the Prophet Muhammad (PBUH) illuminate the divine consequences of animal mistreatment. Islamic law requires the humane slaughter of food animals, thereby minimizing animal suffering.

Addressing Contemporary Environmental Issues: An Islamic Perspective

Today's fast-changing technology and urban sprawl pose new environmental challenges. With its timeless principles, Islam offers insightful and solution-oriented perspectives on modern issues. Climate change, caused by humans, is a major global health issue.

Pollution and waste, especially plastic, are major environmental issues. Due to its environmental impact, some Islamic scholars argue that plastic's widespread use is wasteful under the Qur'anic principle of *Israf* [12]. Islam places great emphasis on *taharah* or cleanliness. Given the prevalence of global pollution, protecting the environment is a religious duty. Modern Muslim communities promote "Eco-Islam," which emphasizes reducing carbon emissions and waste [15, 16].

Islamic leaders and academics also shape Muslim environmental consciousness [17]. Imams worldwide are emphasizing environmental issues in their Friday *khutbah* (sermons). This practice links religious scriptures to environmental issues [18]. Environmental studies and Islamic ethics are being taught in Islamic schools to create environmentally conscious Muslims [19].

Conclusion

Given that environmental health is one of the core competencies of public health, it can be argued that at the heart of Islam lies a profound respect for the environment that is woven into its teachings, practices, and ethical considerations, striving for the greater good of public health. This is not a peripheral theme, but a central tenet, highlighting the intimate relationship between believers and the natural world around them. The Holy Qur'an and the Hadiths of Prophet Muhammad (PBUH) with their myriad of references to nature serve as a perennial guide, urging believers towards responsible environmental stewardship, mindful consumption, and waste minimization. Both the Holy Qur'an and the Prophetic Hadiths could be used as influential sources to promote environmental health beliefs, practices, and principles in Muslim communities and Muslim-majority countries.

Moreover, the environmental ethics espoused by Islam are not exclusive in their relevance. They carry a universal message, emphasizing ecological balance, sustainability, and respect for all living beings – principles that resonate across cultures, faiths, and philosophies. As the world grapples with increasingly pressing environmental challenges, the Islamic perspective offers not only divine wisdom from the past but also contemporary environmental health guidance for the future.

References

1. Schwarte, C. Environmental protection in Islamic law: an overview on potential influences for legal developments in Iraq. *Local Environment*. 2003;8(5):567–76. https://doi.org/10.1080/1354983032000143725

2. Ashtankar, O. Islamic perspectives on environmental protection. *International Journal of Applied Research*. 2016;2 (1):438–41.

3. Aboul-Enein, B. H. "The earth is your mosque": narrative perspectives of environmental health and education in the Holy Quran. *Journal of Environmental Studies and Sciences*. 2018;8(1):22–31. https://doi.org/10.1007/s13412-017-0444-7

4. Rizk, R. R. Islamic environmental ethics. *Journal of Islamic Accounting and Business Research*. 2014;5(2):194–204. https://doi.org/10.1108/JIABR-09-2012-0060

5. Sunan Ibn Majah. *Sunan Ibn Majah 425*. In-book reference: Book 1, Hadith 159. Available from: https://sunnah.com/ibnmajah:425

6. Sahih al-Bukhari. *Sahih al-Bukhari 2320*. In-book reference: Book 41, Hadith 1. Available from: https://sunnah.com/bukhari:2320

7. Sunan an-Nasa'i. *Sunan an-Nasa'i 4446*. In-book reference: Book 43, Hadith 86. Available from: https://sunnah.com/nasai:4446

8. Sunan Abi Dawud. *Sunan Abi Dawud 26*. In-book reference: Book 1, Hadith 26. Available from: https://sunnah.com/abudawud:26

9. Sunan Ibn Majah. *Sunan Ibn Majah 3349*. In-book reference: Book 29, Hadith 99. Available from: https://sunnah.com/ ibnmajah:3349

10. Gada, M. Y. Environmental ethics in Islam: principles and perspectives. *World Journal of Islamic History and Civilization*. 2014;4(4):130–38.

11. Parker, L. Religious environmental education? The new school curriculum in Indonesia. *Environmental Education Research*. 2017;23(9):1249–72. https://doi .org/10.1080/13504622.2016.1150425

12. Muttaqin, Z. The nature of excessive behavior (ISRAF) in the Islamic economic framework. *Journal of Business and Economics Review*. 2019;4(1):49–57. http:// dx.doi.org/10.35609/jber.2019.4.1(6)

13. Mansour, M. S., Hassan, K. H., & Bagheri, P. *Shari'ah* perspective on green jobs and environmental ethics. *Ethics, Policy & Environment*. 2017;20(1):59–77. https:// doi.org/10.1080/21550085.2017.1291829

14. Al-Alawi, A., Sohail, M., Kayaga, S., & Al-Alawi, A. Water management in mosques of Oman. *Sustainable Water Resources Management*. 2021;7:1–10. https://doi .org/10.1007/s40899-021-00581-1

15. Al-Damkhi, A. M. Environmental ethics in Islam: principles, violations, and future perspectives. *International Journal of Environmental Studies*. 2008;65(1):11–31. https://doi.org/10.1080/ 00207230701859724

16. Abdelzaher, D. M., Kotb, A., & Helfaya, A. Eco-Islam: beyond the principles of why and what, and into the principles of how. *Journal of Business Ethics*. 2019;155:623–43. https://doi.org/10.1007/ s10551-017-3518-2

17. Abdelzaher, D. M. & Abdelzaher, A. Beyond environmental regulations: exploring the potential of "eco-Islam" in boosting environmental ethics within SMEs in Arab markets. *Journal of Business Ethics*. 2017;145:357–71. https:// doi.org/10.1007/s10551-015-2833-8

18. Mangunjaya, F. M. & McKay, J. E. Reviving an Islamic approach for environmental conservation in Indonesia. *Worldviews: Global Religions, Culture, and Ecology*. 2012;16(3):286–305. http:// dx.doi.org/10.1163/15685357-01603006

19. Safei, A. A. & Himayaturohmah, E. Development of environmentally friendly culture in the Islamic boarding school through social intervention strategy. *Al-Hayat: Journal of Islamic Education*. 2023;7(1):226–42. https://doi.org/10 .35723/ajie.v7i1.323

Sleep and Health:
An Islamic Perspective

Ahmed S. BaHammam

Introduction

Muslims look to Islam as a way of life, and hence many of them follow the instructions of Islam in all their activities of daily living, including sleep.

Sleep is mentioned frequently in the Qur'an, including in the following verse: "*And among his signs is your sleep by night and by day and your seeking of His bounty. Verily in that are Signs for those who hearken*" (Q Ar-Rum 30:23). Further, Islam has maintained instructions and guidance for followers about the manners of good sleep.

Types of Sleep in the Qur'an

In the Qur'an, sleep is mentioned both using the word "sleep" itself (in Arabic, *Noum*) and using other words that reflect unique definitions or types of sleep. In total, the word "sleep," or some of its synonyms, occurs nine times in the Qur'an. Overall, several Arabic words are used to express sleep in the Qur'an. Generally, however, the various terms for "sleep" refer to different states which essentially correspond to the different sleep stages that we know today:

Sinah: This expression has been described as slumber, or dozing off for a very short time, during which arousal due to any environmental stimulant is prompt, which may correlate with stage 1 sleep. One verse in the Qur'an uses the term *sinah* when describing God (Allah): "*No slumber (Sinah) can seize Him nor sleep*" (Q Al-Baqarah 2:255). In the Qur'an, sleep implies a manifestation of weakness and a bodily need for rest. Therefore, while the Creator (Allah) does not sleep or doze off, His creations, including humankind, need sleep every day.

Nu'aas: Two verses in the Qur'an use the word *nu'aas*. The first, "*Remember when He covered you with a slumber (nu'aas) as a security from him*" (Q Al-Anfal 8:11), describes the fear and stress experienced by those participating in the battle of *Badr* as well as the subsequent relief and feelings of security, which followed a period of slumber (*nu'aas*). In this verse, *nu'aas* refers to a short nap, which may imply a state of sleep deeper than *sinah*. The second verse is as follows: "*Then after the distress, He sent down security upon you. Slumber (nu'aas) overtook a party of you, while, another party was thinking about themselves (as how to save their own selves)*" (Q Al 'Imran 3:154). Current data suggest that short naps could reduce stress and blood pressure, with the most remarkable changes in blood pressure occurring between lights off and sleep onset [1-4].

Ruqood: This word has been deciphered differently among various interpreters of the Qur'an. However, the most appropriate definition in our view is sleep for an extended period, as God has described the people of the Cave (*as'hab al-Kahf*, who are known in Christian literature as "The Seven Sleepers of Ephesus") [5] with this term in the Qur'an [6]: "*And you would have thought them awake, whereas they were asleep (ruqood)*" (Q Al-Kahf 18:18). The Qur'an states the people of the Cave stayed in their Cave for three hundred (solar) years, adding nine (for lunar years) (Q Al-Kahf 18:25) [7].

Hojoo: This term, referring to "sleep at night," appears in the Qur'an, describing the pious believers who fear God (Allah): "*They used to sleep but little by night (hojoo). And in the hours before dawn, they were (found) asking (Allah) for forgiveness*" (Q Adh-Dhaariyaat 51:17–18).

Subaat: The word *subaat* is drawn from the Arabic word *sabt*, which implies disconnecting [6]. Therefore, *subaat* may refer to a disconnection from the nearby environment while asleep. One verse in the Qur'an explains the purpose of sleep: "*And we made your sleep (subaat) as a thing for rest*" (Q An-Naba' 78:9). Therefore, *subaat* may correspond to a deeper state of sleep, in which arousal from sleep is more difficult.

According to the above descriptions, it is reasonable to arrange sleep stages or states into *sinah* and *nu'aas*, followed by *hojoo* and then *subaat*.

Circadian Rhythm

The Qur'an frequently presents day and night among the great signs of the Creator (Allah). The alteration of day and night is mentioned in 37 places in the Qur'an. In the Qur'an, the word "night" always appears before the word "day": "*And We have appointed the night and the day as two signs. Then We have obliterated the sign of the night (with darkness) while We made the sign of the day illuminating*" (Q Al-Israa 17:12). It is evident that the Qur'an deals with humans as diurnal creatures that need light in the daytime and darkness and sleep at night: "*And He it is Who has made the night a garment for you, and sleep a rest. And He has made the day a time of rising to life and going about (for daily livelihood)*" (Q Al-Furqan 25:47). The Qur'an emphasizes the significance of the circadian repetition of light and darkness and counts the succession of night and day as a blessing from Allah:

> Say: See ye? If Allah were to make the Night perpetual over you to the Day of Judgment, what God is there other than Allah, who can give you enlightenment? Will ye not then hearken? Say: See ye? If Allah were to make the Day perpetual over you to the Day of Judgment, what God is there other than Allah, who can give you a Night in which ye can rest? Will ye not then see? It is out of His Mercy that He has made for you Night and Day – that ye may rest therein, and that ye may seek of His Grace – and in order that ye may be grateful.
>
> (Q Al-Qasas 28:71–73)

Muslims pray five mandatory daily prayers. The first prayer (*Fajar*) is at dawn time. Therefore, Muslims are obliged to wake up early every day, on both weekdays and weekends. The final prayer of the day (*Ishaa*) is in the evening time (approximately two hours after sunset), and then there are no obligatory prayers until dawn to allow sleep overnight. Following prayer times strictly influences sleep time and light exposure. Summer nights have earlier dawns and shorter nights; therefore, Muslims may have less sleep during summer nights as they have to wake up for *Fajar* prayer at dawn. A recent study evaluated the effect of waking up for *Fajar* prayer during the summertime on sleep architecture and daytime sleepiness. Results showed that subjects who split sleep due to the *Fajar* prayer had no differences in sleep architecture or daytime sleepiness compared to those who consolidated their sleep (did not wake up for *Fajar* prayer) when the total sleep duration was preserved [8].

Islamic prayer times were originally set according to the movement of the sun. Because of the tilt of the earth, its rotation and revolution around the sun, the various latitudes of the earth's locations, and daylight savings time, prayer times are not fixed and are affected by seasons and locations [9].

Sleep Position

In Islamic culture, certain sleep positions are encouraged while others are discouraged based on the practice (Sunnah) and recommendations of Prophet Muhammad (PBUH). Sleeping on the right side, especially in the early part of sleep when going to bed, is one of the practices of the Prophet (PBUH) that many Muslims try to follow. The Prophet (PBUH) advised, "Whenever you go to bed, perform ablution like that for the prayer, and lie on your right side" [10].

The Prophet (PBUH) told of a man who was lying on his stomach: "Allah and his Prophet dislike this position" [11]. A recent study demonstrated that sleep posture may affect waste removal [12]. This study checked the clearance of waste from the brain, including soluble amyloid β (Aβ). It is known that the glymphatic pathway, which expedites the clearance of waste in the brain, is controlled by the brain's arousal level, whereas, during sleep, the brain's interstitial space volume expands (compared with wakefulness), resulting in faster waste removal [12]. Using fluorescence microscopy and radioactive tracers in rats, the investigators demonstrated that glymphatic transport was lowest in the prone position and most efficient in the lateral position [12].

Naps (*Qailulah*)

Napping is a cross-cultural practice that occurs throughout one's lifespan [13]. A brief midday nap (called *qailulah* in Islamic culture) is an intensely rooted practice in Muslim culture, and for some Muslims, it takes a religious attribute (Sunnah). Prophet Muhammad (PBUH) said, "Take a short nap, for Devils do not take naps" [14]. Another Hadith by Prophet Muhammad (PBUH) presents specifics about nap time, advising, "Sleep at the beginning of the day is stupidity, in the middle of it is (an act of) character, and at the end of it is imbecility" [15]. A third Hadith, narrated in *Sahih Al-Bukhari*, explains, "We used to offer the Jumua (Friday) prayer with the Prophet and then take the afternoon nap" [16]. Friday being considered the weekend is a practice carried out by many Muslims to compensate for the sleep debt during weekdays. In addition, several studies have demonstrated that daytime naps are common in Islamic cultures in different age groups [17–20].

Importance of Sleep

Islam emphasizes the importance of getting enough sleep to protect humans. According to one Hadith by the Prophet (PBUH), "If anyone of you feels drowsy while praying, you should go to bed (sleep) until your slumber is over" [21]. The Prophet (PBUH) told one of his companions (Ibn Amr), who was praying the whole night, "Offer prayers and also sleep at night, as your body has a right on you" [22]. Another Hadith narrates,

Once, the Prophet (PBUH) entered the Mosque and saw a rope hanging between its two pillars. He inquired, "What is this rope?" The people replied, "This rope is for Zainab, who, when she feels tired, holds it (to keep standing for the prayer)." The Prophet (PBUH) said, "Don't use it. Remove the rope. You should pray as long as you feel active, and when you get tired, sleep." [23]

Another Hadith, narrated by Aisha (wife of the Prophet [PBUH]), tells the following story:

A woman from the tribe of Bani Asad was sitting with me, and Allah's Apostle (PBUH) came to my house and said, "Who is this?" I said, "(She is) so-and-so. She does not sleep at night because she is engaged in prayer." The Prophet (PBUH) said disapprovingly, "Do (good) deeds which are within your capacity as Allah never gets tired of giving rewards till you get tired of doing good deeds." [24]

Sleep Manners

There are sleep habits in the Muslim tradition that many Muslims try to perform every night following the practice of the Prophet (PBUH) (Sunnah):

1. **Early bedtime and early rise time**: The Prophet (PBUH) encouraged his companions not to get involved in any activity after *Ishaa* prayer (darkness prayer, which is approximately two hours after sunset). It is narrated that the Prophet (PBUH) said, "One should not sleep before the night prayer, nor have discussions after it" [25]. Furthermore, Muslims are expected to wake up for *Fajar* prayer approximately one hour before sunrise, as the Prophet Muhammad (PBUH) told his companions that God blesses early morning work. Furthermore, Muslims are discouraged from following their prayer with sleep, as the Prophet (PBUH) did not sleep after the *Fajar* prayer [6].

2. **Sleep position**: As previously discussed, sleeping on the right side rather than in the prone position is encouraged.

3. **Biphasic (bimodal) nocturnal sleep pattern**: The Prophet (PBUH) used to retire to bed early at night and get up later for night prayer. It has been narrated that Aisha (wife of Prophet Muhammad), when asked about the night prayer of the Prophet (PBUH), answered, "He used to sleep early at night and get up in its last part to pray, and then return to his bed. When the Mu'adh-dhin pronounced the Adhan (for dawn prayer), he would get up. If he was in need of a bath he would take it; otherwise, he would perform ablution and then go out (for the prayer)" [26]. Some Muslims were following this biphasic nocturnal sleep before the preindustrial era [27]. In a description of sleep obtained by residents of Muscat, Oman in the early nineteenth century, they were said to retire early to rest, lying down before 10 o'clock (except when on a journey, or at sea), so that before midnight their first sleep was usually over [28].

4. **Yawning**: Yawning is not acceptable behavior among Muslims, especially in public places. If yawning occurs, the yawner is instructed to cover their mouth with their hand. The Prophet (PBUH) said, "Yawning is from Satan. If you are about to yawn, you should try to stop it as much as possible. If you yawn, Satan will laugh" [29].

Conclusion

In general, sleep is considered one of the signs of the greatness of Allah (God) in the Islamic faith, and Muslims are urged to investigate this important sign. We urge health and social science researchers who are interested in sleep to investigate culturally congruent religious sources to comprehend older civilizations' ideas, behaviors, and practices concerning sleep and sleep disorders.

References

1. Naska, A., Oikonomou, E., Trichopoulou, A., Psaltopoulou, T., & Trichopoulos, D. Siesta in healthy adults and coronary mortality in the general population. *Archives of Internal Medicine.* 2007;167 (3):296–301. https://doi.org/10.1001/archinte.167.3.296

2. Zaregarizi, M., Edwards, B., George, K., Harrison, Y., Jones, H., & Atkinson, G. Acute changes in cardiovascular function during the onset period of daytime sleep: comparison to lying awake and standing. *Journal of Applied Physiology.* 2007;103 (4):1332–38. https://doi.org/10.1152/japplphysiol.00474.2007

3. Brindle, R. C. & Conklin, S. M. Daytime sleep accelerates cardiovascular recovery after psychological stress. *International Journal of Behavioral Medicine.* 2011;19 (1):111–14. https://doi.org/10.1007/s12529-011-9150-0

4. Oriyama, S., Miyakoshi, Y., & Kobayashi, T. Effects of two 15-min naps on the subjective sleepiness, fatigue and heart rate variability of night shift nurses. *Industrial Health.* 2014;52(1):25–35. https://doi.org/10.2486/indhealth.2013-0043

5. Leaman, O., ed. *The Qur'an: An Encyclopedia.* London: Routledge. 2006.

6. Al-Abid Zuhd, E. The miracle verses and its impact about sleeping in Qur'an. *Aljameah Alislamiah Journal.* 2010;18 (2):50–215.

7. Al-Qurtubī. Tafsir Al-Qurtubī: Islam Port. [online]. [Accessed November 2, 2021]. Available from: https://islamport.com/

8. Bahammam, A. S., Sharif, M. M., Spence, D. W., & Pandi-Perumal, S. R. Sleep architecture of consolidated and split sleep due to the dawn (*Fajr*) prayer among Muslims and its impact on daytime sleepiness. *Annals of Thoracic Medicine.* 2012;7(1):36–41. https://doi.org/10.4103/1817-1737.91560

9. Raisal, A. Y. & Rakhmadi, A. J. Understanding the effect of revolution and rotation of the earth on prayer times using accurate times. *Ulul Albab Jurnal Studi dan Penelitian Hukum Islam.* 2020;4 (1):81–101. http://dx.doi.org/10.30659/jua.v4i1.10936

10. Sahih al-Bukhari. *Sahih al-Bukhari 247.* In-book reference: Book 4, Hadith 113. Available from: https://sunnah.com/bukhari:247

11. Jami' at-Tirmidhi. *Jami' at-Tirmidhi 2768.* In-book reference: Book 43, Hadith 38. Available from: https://sunnah.com/tirmidhi:2768

12. Lee, H., Xie, L., Yu, M., Kang, H., Feng, T., Deane, R., et al. The effect of body posture on brain glymphatic transport. *The Journal of Neuroscience: The Official Journal of the Society for Neuroscience.* 2015;35(31):11034–44. https://doi.org/10.1523/jneurosci.1625-15.2015

13. Milner, C. E. & Cote, K. A. Benefits of napping in healthy adults: impact of nap length, time of day, age, and experience with napping. *Journal of Sleep Research.* 2009;18(2):272–81. https://doi.org/10.1111/j.1365-2869.2008.00718.x

14. Albani, M. N. D. *Sahih al-jami' al-saghir wa-ziyadatah (al-Fath al-kabir).* Beirut: al-Maktab al-Islami. 1969.

15. Al-Adab Al-Mufrad. *Al-Adab Al-Mufrad 1242.* In-book reference: Book 52, Hadith 5. Available from: https://sunnah.com/adab:1242

16. Sahih al-Bukhari. *Sahih al-Bukhari 941.* In-book reference: Book 11, Hadith 65. Available from: https://sunnah.com/ bukhari:941

17. BaHammam, A. S. Sleep pattern, daytime sleepiness, and eating habits during the month of Ramadan. *Sleep and Hypnosis.* 2003;5(4):165–72.

18. BaHammam, A. S., AlFaris, E., Shaikh, S., & Bin Saeed, A. Prevalence of sleep problems and habits in a sample of Saudi primary school children. *Annals of Saudi Medicine.* 2006;26(1):7–13. https://doi .org/10.5144/0256-4947.2006.7

19. Wali, S. O., Krayem, A. B., Samman, Y. S., Mirdad, S., Alshimemeri, A. A., & Almobaireek, A. Sleep disorders in Saudi health care workers. *Annals of Saudi Medicine.* 1999;19(5):406–9. https://doi .org/10.5144/0256-4947.1999.406

20. BaHammam, A. S., Alghannam, A. F., Aljaloud, K. S., Aljuraiban, G. S., AlMarzooqi, M. A., Dobia, A. M., et al. Joint consensus statement of the Saudi Public Health Authority on the recommended amount of physical activity, sedentary behavior, and sleep duration for healthy Saudis: background, methodology, and discussion. *Annals of Thoracic Medicine.* 2021;16(3):225–38. https://doi.org/10.4103/atm.atm_32_21

21. Sahih al-Bukhari. *Sahih al-Bukhari 212.* In-book reference: Book 4, Hadith 78. Available from: https://sunnah.com/ bukhari:212

22. Sahih al-Bukhari. *Sahih al-Bukhari 5199.* In-book reference: Book 67, Hadith 133. Available from: https://sunnah.com/ bukhari:5199

23. Sahih al-Bukhari. *Sahih al-Bukhari 1150.* In-book reference: Book 19, Hadith 31. Available from: https://sunnah.com/ bukhari:1150

24. Sahih al-Bukhari. *Sahih al-Bukhari 1151.* In-book reference: Book 19, Hadith 32. Available from: https://sunnah.com/ bukhari:1151

25. Sahih al-Bukhari. *Sahih al-Bukhari 568.* In-book reference: Book 9, Hadith 45. Available from: https://sunnah.com/ bukhari:568

26. Sahih al-Bukhari. *Sahih al-Bukhari 1146.* In-book reference: Book 19, Hadith 27. Available from: https://sunnah.com/ bukhari:1146

27. Ekirch, A. R. Segmented sleep in preindustrial societies. *Sleep.* 2016;39 (3):715–16. https://doi.org/10.5665/sleep .5558

28. Shaik, M. *History of Seyd Said, Sultan of Muscat: Together with an Account of the Countries and People on the Shores of the Persian Gulf, Particularly of the Wahabees.* London: John Booth. 1819.

29. Sahih al-Bukhari. *Sahih al-Bukhari 3289.* In-book reference: Book 59, Hadith 98. Available from: https://sunnah.com/ bukhari:3289

Addictive Behaviors and Public Health

G. Hussein Rassool

Introduction

It can be argued that modern secular society has an appetite for intoxicating substances and activities that give rise to addictive behaviors. The use of psychoactive substances (whether legal, illegal, or prescribed) continues to be a major public health problem. The harms caused by alcohol and drugs include physical, psychological, social, economic, and spiritual harm as well as environmental damage. The harms that result from the association between substance use and mental health problems are of special concern as suicide is strongly related to psychiatric disorders and comorbid substance abuse, particularly with alcohol use disorders [1]. There is a dearth of research on the prevalence of alcohol and drug use among the Muslim communities as the "prevalence of alcohol and drug use/abuse among Muslims is extremely difficult to determine as it relies upon self-reporting a stigmatized behavior" [2 p. 20]. The world's lowest levels of alcohol consumption are found in Muslim-majority countries. While alcohol consumption is ostensibly forbidden and alcohol and Islam are generally considered to be mutually exclusive, some Muslims do consume alcohol.

The types of psychoactive substances used by Muslims are no different than non-Muslim populations. Muslims use opiates, cannabis and its resin, crystalline methamphetamine, khat, and fenetylline (Captagon). Khat is also a psychostimulant. Khat refers to the young and tender leaves and shoots of the khat tree (*Catha edulis*). Khat has many names including "qat" (Yemen), "jad" or "chad" (Ethiopia and Somalia), "miraa" (Kenya), or "marungi" (Uganda and Rwanda). Captagon was first created as an alternative to amphetamine and methamphetamine and was used to treat attention deficit hyperactivity disorder and, less commonly, depression.

Opium smoking is a traditional practice in the Islamic Republic of Iran, Pakistan, and Afghanistan, resulting in a high prevalence of opiate use and intravenous drug use with increasing prevalence of HIV infection [3]. This chapter aims to examine addictive behaviors from an Islamic perspective and provide a critical review of the public health approach (abstinence and harm-reduction) in addictive behaviors.

Islamic Perspective on Addiction

Despite an array of studies that have hailed moderate alcohol use for its health benefits including reduced likelihood of cardiovascular diseases and all-cause mortality, these benefits may have been overestimated [4]. There is a paradox whereby there may be limited benefits but overall there are more psychosocial, economic, environmental, and spiritual harms. In relation to drinking alcohol while pregnant, it has been recommended that the safest approach is not to drink alcohol at all to keep risks to the baby at a minimum due to the fetal alcohol syndrome that affects newborn babies when the mother is exposed to alcohol during her pregnancy [5]. Regardless of the findings on the use of alcohol as a social lubricant, Islam takes a strong prohibitive and preventive stance and forbids all intoxicants (alcohol, drugs, and tobacco), regardless of the quantity or kind, because any substance that harms the body is prohibited. Allah mentions in the Qur'an, "*They ask you about wine and gambling. Say: In them is great sin and [yet, some] benefit for people. However, their sin is greater than their benefit. And they ask you what they should spend. Say: The excess [beyond needs]. Thus, Allah makes clear to you the verses [of revelation] that you might give thought to*" (Q Al-Baqarah 2:219). In this verse, the Qur'an acknowledges that there may be some benefits in consuming alcohol, but the potential harms outweigh any benefits. Modern scholars have used the principles of Islamic jurisprudence to derive judgments regarding many of the illicit drugs available today that were unknown at the time of the revelation of the Qur'an. Therefore, the prohibition has been extended to refer to any recreational drug with similar qualities, including cocaine, methamphetamines, heroin, cannabis, and other substances. In another passage, Allah mentions in the Qur'an,

> O you who have believed, indeed, intoxicants, gambling, [sacrificing on] stone alters [to other than Allah], and divining arrows are but defilement from the work of Satan, so avoid it that you may be successful. Satan only wants to cause between you animosity and hatred through intoxicants and gambling and to avert you from the remembrance of Allah and from prayer. So, will you not desist?

(Q Al-Ma'idah 5:90–91)

In an exegesis of the fourteenth-century Arab historian, Ibn Kathir, he stated that Allah forbids His believing servants from consuming *khamr* and from *maysir*, or gambling [6]. This suggests that addictive behaviors are extended to include gambling in addition to the use of alcohol and drugs (psychoactive substances, tobacco, and *shisha* smoking). This is echoed in the statement made by Philips [7]. The term used in these two verses, *khamr*, refers to all forms of intoxicating drugs, as Prophet Muhammad (PBUH) stated: "Every intoxicant is *khamr* (wine) and every *khamr* is unlawful" [8]. It was narrated that 'Aisha was asked about drinks and she said, "The Messenger of Allah (PBUH) used to forbid all intoxicants" [9]. It was also narrated that Ibn Sirin said, "A man came to Ibn 'Umar and said: 'Our families make drinks for us by soaking (fruits) at night, and in the morning we drink them.' He said: 'I forbid you to drink intoxicants whether in small amounts or large. May Allah bear witness that I forbid you to drink intoxicants whether in small amounts or large'" [10]. The Prophet (PBUH) said, "All drinks that produce intoxication are *haram* (forbidden)" [11].

If a substance intoxicates when taken in large quantities, then even small quantities of it are forbidden. Shaykh Yusuf al-Qaradawi stated that the first declaration made by the Prophet (PBUH) concerning this matter said that not only is *khamr* (wine or alcohol) prohibited but that the definition of *khamr* extends to any substance that intoxicates, in whatever form or under whatever name it may appear [12]. Drugs such as marijuana, cocaine, opium, and the like are included in the prohibited category of *khamr* [12]. Abu Bakr bin 'Abdur-Rahman bin Al-Harith narrated that his father said, "I heard 'Uthman say: 'Avoid *khamr* for it is the mother of all evils'" [13]. By labelling drugs and gambling as harmful in the verses of the Qur'an, Allah addresses the natural inclination of human psychology to avoid what causes more harm than benefits. Like alcohol and drugs, the harms of gambling include physical, psychological, emotional, and financial problems. Philips stated that by classifying drugs on par with games of chance, idolatrous practices, and fortune-telling, all of which have been pronounced as forbidden, the prohibition of drugs is further emphasized [7]. He further suggested that God (Allah) identified the origin of drugs for humans to realize that they are weapons of their most avowed enemy, Satan. In the battle for human souls, Satan uses a variety of tools which he beautifies and makes alluring to trap human beings [7].

In effect, anything that takes away their senses and obstructs a Muslim person from remembering Allah in ritual players is discouraged. In addition, the individual may lose their moral compass and indulge in deviant or immoral behaviors. It can also be inferred from the aforementioned Qur'anic verses that "Allah addresses the human psyche by promising success to those who avoid intoxicants … the social benefits to both the individual and family are even more priceless" [7]. The verse of the Qur'an "*So will you not desist?*" (Q Al-Ma'idah 5:91) concludes with a rhetorical question. This question is addressed to those who can contemplate or reflect on this verse and appeal to their reasoning and common sense to abstain from the evils of alcohol, drugs, and gambling.

Prevention and Public Health

Islam established a zero-tolerance policy towards addictions. The public health approach in the response to addiction began in the seventh century during the first Islamic caliphate. Allah says in the Qur'an, "*And let there be [arising] from you a nation inviting to [all that is] good, enjoining what is right and forbidding what is wrong, and those will be successful*" (Q Al 'Imran 3:104). One of the principles of Islamic jurisprudence known as *sadd al-dhara'i* provides a good example of the importance of primary prevention in Islam. Kamali stated,

> The whole concept of *sadd al-dhara'i* is founded in the idea of preventing an "evil" before it materializes. It is therefore not always necessary that the result should take place. It is rather the objective expectation that a means is likely to lead to an evil result that renders the means in question unlawful even without the realization of the expected result." [14 p. 268]

The model that Islam adopted in tackling alcohol and drugs is based on prohibition and prevention leading to the total abstinence model – also known as the 12-step faith-based model. The Islamic model of the 12-step recovery program is the service provided, for example, by the Millati Islami. Millati Islami is a fellowship of men and women who look to Allah (God) to guide them on Millati Islami (the Path of Peace). While recovering, they strive to become rightly guided Muslims, submitting their will and services to Allah [15]. In contrast to the abstinence model, due to the increased use of drugs and injecting behavior (and the control of HIV), harm reduction approaches have been proposed. Harm reduction programs include providing information about safer drug use and safer sex, needle exchange schemes (pharmacy-based needle exchange or other forms of needle exchange), programs to reduce the risk associated with HIV and hepatitis, and the supervision of the consumption of methadone or other opiate substitutes. Regarding the control of the HIV pandemic, evidence suggests that harm reduction approaches had some success in the Islamic Republic of Iran [16, 17], Malaysia [18], and

Indonesia [19] where both needle exchange programs and opioid substitution therapy have been implemented. However, regions in the Middle East and North Africa (MENA) have not adopted the harm reduction approach. It is reported that only 9 of 19 nations there have employed any sort of harm reduction program. Looking at the Middle East alone, that ratio becomes even weaker. Two of the three nations that shut down OAT (opioid agonist therapies) programs in the last year include Bahrain and Kuwait [20].

Many Islamic countries do not support the policy and practice of harm reduction despite the nature and extent of drug misuse and HIV epidemics in Islamic countries such as Iran which are driven by intravenous drug use. Political, social, cultural, and religious factors complicate the implementation of harm reduction in the Islamic world. It has been argued that the implementation of harm reduction in the MENA region will likely depend on finding ways to communicate its ideas in theologically and culturally sensitive ways [20]. The main contention is that religious and political leaders have traditionally opposed harm reduction approaches on the basis that the distribution of needles and condoms would encourage and imply acceptance of drug use and illegal sexual relations and that opioid substitution therapy would compromise the national goal to become drug-free [18, 21]. This means that harm reduction approaches are alien to Islamic beliefs and practices and, thus, cannot be applied as acceptable strategies. Madani has suggested the strategies to prevent HIV infection in Islamic countries should include strengthening both Islamic and health education; encouraging people to follow and implement the Islamic principles and values that forbid adultery, homosexuality, and intravenous drug use; and promoting the practice of safe sex only through legal marriage [22].

In Islamic countries, advocates of harm reduction approaches to control the drug-driven HIV epidemics based their arguments on the *Maqasid al-Shariah* (Higher Objectives of Islam). These principles are the preservation and protection of faith, life, intellect, progeny, and wealth. According to Kamarulzaman and Saifuddeen, "Harm reduction programs are permissible and in fact provide a practical solution to a problem that could result in far greater damage to the society at large if left unaddressed" [23 p. 115]. Moreover, the authors found that the principle of injury in Islam asserts that "no one should be hurt or cause hurt to others" [23 p. 116]. This applies the maxim of the "lesser of the two evils" principle that is used to justify the permissibility of harm reduction approaches to drug use and HIV that pertain to matters of life and death. Another principle is "the necessity to overrule the prohibition in situations where there is great need, thereby rendering something that is originally prohibited to become permissible" [23 p. 116]. Q Al-Baqarah 2:173 asserts this principle: "*He has only forbidden to you dead animals, blood, the flesh of swine, and that which has been dedicated to other than God. But whoever is forced [by necessity], neither desiring [it] nor transgressing [its limit], there is no sin upon him. Indeed, God is Forgiving and Merciful.*" Other principles state that "harm must be treated and benefits must be brought forth" and "public interest should be given priority over personal interest" [23 p. 117].

Conclusion

The above principles have been used to implement harm reduction approaches in a few Islamic countries. There are a plurality of norms and public policies concerning alcohol and both licit and illicit drug use in Muslim communities. Islam takes a strong prohibitive and preventive stance in the public health challenges involving drugs, alcohol, and gambling activities and forbids all intoxicants (alcohol, drugs, and tobacco) regardless of the quantity or type. The dominant approach to Islamic-based public health is based on a unified standard approach to abstinence and primary prevention. However, a few Muslim-majority countries have adopted the harm reduction approach in public health policy.

References

1. Schneider, B. Substance use disorders and risk for completed suicide. *Archives of Suicide Research*. 2009;13(4):303–16. https://doi.org/10.1080/13811110903263191

2. Arfken, C. & Ahmed, S. Ten years of substance use research in Muslim populations: where do we go from here? *Journal of Muslim Mental Health*. 2016;10 (1):13–24. https://doi.org/10.3998/jmmh .10381607.0010.103

3. UNODC. World drug report 2020. [online]. 2020 [Accessed March 22, 2023]. Available from: https://wdr.unodc.org/ wdr2020/index2020.html

4. Knott, G. S., Coombs, N., Stamatakis, E., & Biddulph, J. P. All cause mortality and the case for age specific alcohol consumption guidelines: pooled analyses of up to 10 population based cohorts. *BMJ*. 2015;350:h384. https://doi.org/10 .1136/bmj.h384

5. NHS UK. Drinking alcohol while pregnant. [online]. 2017 [Accessed March 22, 2023]. Available from: www .nhs.uk/conditions/pregnancy-and-baby/ alcohol-medicines-drugs-pregnant/? tabname=getting-pregnant

6. Kathir, I. Abualrub, J., Khitab, N., Khitab, H., Walker, A., Al-Jibali, M., & Ayoub, S., Trans. *Tafsir ibn Kathir*. Saudi Arabia: Darussalam Publishers and Distributors. 2000.

7. Philips, A. B. *War on Drugs Began 14 Centuries Ago*. 2008. Available from: https://d1.Islamhouse.com/data/en/ih_ articles/single/en_War_on_drugs.pdf

8. Sunan Ibn Majah. *Sunan Ibn Majah 3390*. In-book reference: Book 30, Hadith 20. Available from: https://sunnah.com/ ibnmajah:3390

9. Sunan an-Nasa'i. *Sunan an-Nasa'i 5682*. In-book reference: Book 51, Hadith 144. Available from: https://sunnah.com/ nasai:5682

10. Sunan an-Nasa'i. *Sunan an-Nasa'i 5581*. In-book reference: Book 51, Hadith 43. Available from: https://sunnah.com/ nasai:5581

11. Sahih al-Bukhari. *Sahih al-Bukhari 242*. In-book reference: Book 4, Hadith 108. Available from: https://sunnah.com/ bukhari:242

12. Al-Qaradawi, Y. *The Lawful and the Prohibited in Islam (Al-Halal Wal Haram Fil Islam)*. Oak Brook, IL: American Trust Publications. 1999.

13. Sunan an-Nasa'i. *Sunan an-Nasa'i 5667*. In-book reference: Book 51, Hadith 129. Available from: https://sunnah.com/ nasai:5667

14. Kamali, M. H. *Principles of Islamic Jurisprudence*. Cambridge: Islamic Texts Society. 2006.

15. Millati Islami. Home. [online]. n.d. [Accessed March 22, 2023]. Available from: https://www.millatiislami.org/

16. Nissaramanesh, B., Trace, M., & Roberts, M. *The rise of harm reduction in the Islamic Republic of Iran*. The Beckley Foundation Drug Policy Programme (BFDPP). 2005. Available from: https://carrythemessage.com/ include/iran/2005-07-the-rise-of-harm- reduction-in-the-islamic-republic-of-iran .pdf

17. Razzaghi, E., Nassirimanesh, B., Afshar, P., Ohiri, K., Claeson, M., & Power, R. HIV/AIDS harm reduction in Iran. *The*

Lancet. 2006;368(9534):434–35. https://doi.org/10.1016/S0140-6736(06)69132-0

18. Reid, G. A. & Kamarulzaman, S. K. Malaysia and harm reduction: the challenges and responses. *International Journal of Drug Policy.* 2007;18 (2):136–40. https://doi.org/10.1016/j.drugpo.2006.12.015

19. Mesquita, F., Winsarno, I., Atmosukarto, I. I., Eka, B., Nevendorff, I., Rahmah, A., et al. Public health the leading force of the Indonesian response to the HIV/AIDS crisis among people who inject drugs. *Harm Reduction Journal.* 2007;4(1):9. https://doi.org/10.1186/1477-7517-4-9

20. Fleming, R. Major report assesses the global state of harm reduction. [online]. Filter. 2020 [Accessed March 22, 2023]. Available from: https://filtermag.org/harm-reduction-worldwide/

21. Todd, C. S., Nassiramanesh, B., Stanekzai, M. R., & Kamarulzaman, A. Emerging HIV epidemics in Muslim countries: assessment of different cultural responses to harm reduction and implications for HIV control. *Current HIV/AIDS Reports.* 2007;4(4):151–57. https://doi.org/10.1007/s11904-007-0022-9

22. Madani, T. A., Al-Mazrou, Y. Y., Al-Jeffri, M. H., & Al Huzaim, N. S. Epidemiology of the human immunodeficiency virus in Saudi Arabia: 18-year surveillance results and prevention from an Islamic perspective. *BMC Infectious Diseases.* 2004;4:25. https://doi.org/10.1186/1471-2334-4-25

23. Kamarulzaman, A. & Saifuddeen, S. M. Islam and harm reduction. *International Journal of Drug Policy.* 2010;21 (2):115–18. https://doi.org/10.1016/j.drugpo.2009.11.003

Highlighting the Concepts, Principles, and Values of Communication: A Brief Islamic Perspective

Amal I. Khalil

Introduction

In Islam, interpersonal communication is highly valued for fostering understanding, trust, cooperation, and collaboration among Muslims. It is guided by principles of ethics, morality, respect, justice, forgiveness, and consultation [1]. Prophet Muhammad's (PBUH) examples in the Qur'an and Hadith serve as a guide for Muslims on effective and respectful communication [2]. Islamic teachings emphasize the importance of active listening and empathy towards others. Cultural differences are considered, and Muslims are encouraged to be mindful of these differences in their communication [3]. Additionally, Islamic communication principles address the challenges of globalization and recognize the role of communication technologies in Islamic revitalization [4].

The Origin of Language in the Prospect of Islam

Language communication plays a significant role in Islam, being viewed as a divine gift from Allah. The Arabic language, as the language of the Qur'an, holds particular importance within Islam [5]. Islamic scholars have explored the origins of language, proposing that it emerged as a result of human necessity and social interaction [5]. The Qur'an is considered a communication miracle in Islam, written in Arabic and believed to be the literal word of Allah. Its language is seen as powerful and transformative, capable of impacting believers and nonbelievers alike [5].

Communication Miracles of the Holy Qur'an

The Holy Qur'an is considered to be a communication miracle due to its literary excellence, linguistic beauty, and guidance for humanity. It is believed to be the direct word of Allah revealed to Prophet Muhammad (PBUH) through the Angel Gabriel [6]. The Qur'an effectively communicates complex ideas through simple and relatable language, utilizing literary devices such as metaphor and analogy [7]. It is designed to be easily remembered and recited, emphasizing the importance of clear and straightforward communication [6]. The Qur'an also promotes effective communication by encouraging dialogue, understanding, and the seeking of knowledge from diverse perspectives [7]. Its ability to inspire and motivate people towards righteousness and excellence has had a profound impact on human history and culture [6].

Theoretical Perspectives on Islamic Communication

Islamic scholars and communication researchers have developed theoretical perspectives on Islamic communication to understand its dynamics and impact on behavior. These perspectives include Tawhid, *Adab*, and *Mizan*. Tawhid emphasizes the unity of Allah and suggests that all communication should be directed towards maintaining harmony with Allah, as mentioned in Q Al-An'am 6:162 [8]. *Adab* focuses on proper conduct and behavior in interactions with others, as exemplified by the guidance of Prophet Muhammad (PBUH) to speak good or remain silent [9]. *Mizan* promotes balance and moderation in actions and interactions, supported by the Qur'an's encouragement to maintain a just and balanced community, as stated in Q Al-Baqarah 2:143 [10]. These perspectives provide a framework for understanding Islamic communication and its influence on individual and social behavior.

The Islamic Communication Model

The Islamic communication model encompasses key principles such as Tawhid, *Adab*, sincerity and truthfulness, effective listening, wisdom and *hikmah*, constructive criticism and advice, respect for privacy and confidentiality, and nonverbal communication. Tawhid emphasizes promoting unity and harmony with Allah [6]. *Adab* emphasizes good manners, empathy, and fairness [7]. Sincerity and truthfulness in expression are valued, while effective listening and understanding others' perspectives are important. In Islam, wisdom or *hikmah* guides communication for effective and harmonious interaction. Constructive criticism and advice are encouraged with kindness. Respect for privacy and confidentiality is emphasized, along with modest nonverbal communication [10].

Communication Styles and Principles of Prophet Muhammad (PBUH)

Prophet Muhammad (PBUH) serves as the quintessential role model for Muslims in all aspects of life, including communication. His communication skills were characterized by honesty, clarity, empathy, and active listening [11]. The Qur'an mentions that some referred to him as "an ear," highlighting his attentive listening ability [11]. This communication style of Prophet Muhammad (PBUH) is exemplified in the Qur'an in Q At-Tawbah 9:61. While there may not be a specific verse solely focused on the Prophet's (PBUH) listening skills, the Qur'an and Hadith literature collectively depict his communication style as one characterized by active listening and genuine concern for others [11]. Additionally, he used simple and clear language to convey his message, making it accessible and easy to understand for his audience [12].

Levels of Communication and Social Relationship in Islam

In Islam, communication and social relationships hold significant value and are guided by principles and guidelines at different levels.

Individual Level: Islamic communication emphasizes self-reflection and introspection. Muslims are encouraged to regularly reflect on their thoughts, words, and actions to ensure alignment with Islamic values [12].

Interpersonal Level: Islamic communication focuses on fostering positive relationships based on trust, respect, and empathy. Muslims are encouraged to engage in active listening, demonstrate patience and kindness, and refrain from gossip or negative speech about others [12].

Community Level: Islamic communication highlights social responsibility and civic engagement. Muslims are encouraged to work collectively to promote social justice, support vulnerable community members, and build connections with people of diverse faiths and backgrounds [11].

Global level: Islam emphasizes fostering connections and understanding between diverse cultures and societies across the world. Muslims are encouraged to engage in constructive dialogue with individuals of different faiths, nationalities, and backgrounds to promote mutual understanding, respect, and a more peaceful world [12]. The Qur'an states, "*O mankind! We created you from a single (pair) of a male and a female, and made you into nations and tribes, that you may know each other (not that you may despise each other). Verily, the most honored of you in the sight of Allah is the most righteous of you. And Allah has full knowledge and is well acquainted with all things*" (Q Al-Hujuraat 49:13). This verse emphasizes the importance of acknowledging and appreciating diversity and highlights that righteousness is the true measure of honor. By embracing this perspective, Islamic communication aims to bridge cultural divides and promote harmonious coexistence.

Intercultural Communication and Islamic Principles

Islamic teachings emphasize respect, empathy, and understanding in intercultural communication. Muslims are encouraged to approach people of other cultures with an open mind and seek to understand their perspectives and beliefs [13]. Qur'anic verses such as Q Al-Hujuraat 49:13 highlight the purpose of diversity in fostering knowledge and understanding among humanity. Q Al-Kaafiroon 109:6 emphasizes acceptance of different religious beliefs and promotes respect and tolerance [13]. Islamic principles also emphasize maintaining cultural identity while engaging in intercultural communication, as seen in verses like Q Al-Mumtahanah 60:8 and Q Al-Hujuraat 49:11 [13]. Muslims are encouraged to be advocates of their Islamic heritage and share their culture positively [13]. The Qur'an advises against arrogance and superiority in intercultural communication, as shown in verses like Q Luqmaan 31:19 and Q Al-Israa 17:37 [13].

Islamic Principles and Values of Human Interaction

Islam guides how humans should interact with one another based on principles such as respect, justice, forgiveness, and consultation. These principles promote ethical and moral behavior in human interaction and help to build strong relationships between individuals and communities [14]. The Qur'an states,

> So by mercy from Allah, [O Muhammad], you were lenient with them. And if you had been rude [in speech] and harsh in heart, they would have disbanded from about you. So, pardon them and ask forgiveness for them and consult them in the matter. And when you have decided, then rely upon Allah. Indeed, Allah loves those who rely [upon Him].
>
> (Q Al 'Imran 3:159)

This verse highlights the significance of adopting a compassionate and forgiving attitude towards others [15].

Communication and the Muslim Family

In Muslim families, there is a strong emphasis on family ties and the role of parents in raising children. Parents are responsible for instilling Islamic values and principles in their children from a young age. Communication within the family is based on mutual respect and support, with parents serving as role models [16]. Parents use stories from the Qur'an and the Prophet's (PBUH) life to teach children important lessons about morality and ethics. Examples include the story of Prophet Yusuf (Joseph), which teaches honesty, patience, and forgiveness, and the story of Prophet Ibrahim (Abraham), which teaches obedience, sacrifice, and submission to Allah [17]. The story of Prophet Muhammad (PBUH) emphasizes compassion, kindness, and fairness, as seen in the Conquest of Makkah where the Prophet (PBUH) forgave his former enemies and embraced them with affection and mercy [17].

During adolescence and young adulthood, communication among Muslims becomes more complex as individuals develop their own identities and beliefs. Muslim families typically promote open communication and encourage their children to express themselves and be inquisitive [16, 18, 19]. Parents often play a supportive role in helping their children navigate the challenges of this stage.

Respecting and showing compassion towards the elderly is highly emphasized in Muslim families. The Prophet Muhammad (PBUH) said, "He is not one of us who does not have mercy on our young and does not respect our elders" [1]. This Hadith, narrated by Abu Dawood and At-Tirmidhi, highlights the significance of valuing and caring for both the young and the elderly [19]. In line with this teaching, Muslim families place great importance on providing support and care for their elderly family members. It involves demonstrating respect for their life experiences, wisdom, and civic contributions. This includes actively listening to their stories, seeking their advice, and honoring their opinions. By doing so, Muslim families create an environment where the elderly feel valued, respected, and included in the family dynamics.

Social Media, Globalization, and Islamic Principles

While there are no specific references to social media in primary Islamic sources such as the Holy Qur'an and Prophetic guidance, contemporary Islamic scholars provide modern guidance on responsible and ethical behavior within the context of communication through technology. The concept of *Ihsan* encourages Muslims to embody excellence in behavior and intentions, promoting honesty, kindness, and integrity in their online interactions [20]. Islam also emphasizes the protection of privacy and warns against backbiting and slander. Muslims are advised to be cautious about what they share on social media and to avoid engaging in gossip or spreading rumors. The Qur'anic principle of "enjoining good and forbidding wrong" encourages Muslims to use social media platforms to promote virtue and justice and to speak out against injustice and wrongdoing. Islam encourages responsible and ethical use of social media, with a focus on upholding Islamic values and contributing to the improvement of society through positive online presence [21].

The effects of globalization and communication technologies on Islamic culture are complex and multifaceted. Globalization has led to the spread of Islamic ideas, values, and practices to different parts of the world, increasing the diversity and richness of Islamic culture [22]. However, globalization has also led to the homogenization and commodification of Islamic culture, reducing it to a superficial and commercialized form [23]. Communication technologies have had both positive and negative effects on Islamic culture. On the positive side, these technologies have provided opportunities for Muslims to connect, share ideas, and engage civically and politically [24]. However, they have also facilitated the spread of extremist ideologies, leading to violence and conflict in some regions, which are contrary to Islamic principles [25].

Muslims face challenges in a globalized world, including the influence of globalization and communication technologies on Islamic culture. Despite these challenges, there are opportunities for Muslims to adapt and thrive while adhering to their Islamic values and traditions.

When it comes to individuals with intellectual disabilities, effective communication may require additional support and accommodation, such as visual aids or assistive technology. Islam emphasizes patience and understanding when communicating with those who have difficulty expressing themselves or understanding others. Islamic teachings also stress the importance of inclusion and equity in communication, ensuring that all individuals have access to education and resources that promote understanding, regardless of their abilities or backgrounds [26, 27].

Conclusion

Communication is an important aspect of Islamic principles and values. Since communication serves as the central function in developing a trusting and therapeutic relationship in any health setting, it could be argued that the fundamental constructs of Islamic-based communication promote and uphold the contemporary patient-centered approach. Given that health outcomes depend on successful and effective communication, this chapter offers public health practitioners and educators a culturally congruent form of interaction with Muslim communities around the world. Despite the challenges of globalization in communication technologies today, effective communication for Muslims should involve mutual respect, empathy, honesty, active listening, and mutual understanding.

References

1. Khalil, A. E. The Islamic perspective of interpersonal communication. *Journal of Islamic Studies and Culture*. 2016;4 (2):22–37.

2. Ismail, N., Makhsin, M., Abd Rahim, S. I., Abd Ghani, B., & Rosaidi, N. A. Interpersonal communication skill and *Da'wah Fardiyah* approach in sustainable Islamic spiritual mentoring. In: Kaur, N. & Ahmad, M., eds. *Charting a Sustainable Future of ASEAN in Business and Social* *Sciences*. Singapore: Springer. 2020. 79–86.

3. Yousefzadeh, H. The Islamic basis for mutual understanding in intercultural communication. *Kom casopis za religijske nauke*. 2018;7(3):47–67. http://dx.doi.org/10.5937/kom1802047Y

4. Ali, J. A. Introduction to special issue: Islamic revivalism and social transformation in the modern world. *Religions*. 2023;14:899. https://doi.org/10.3390/rel14070899

5. Khaldun, I. Dowood, N. J., ed. Rosenthal, F., trans. *The Muqaddimah: An Introduction to History.* Princeton, NJ: Princeton University Press. 1967.

6. Li, Z. W. Islamic civilization and the world. *Asian Arabization Journal, Center for Research and Knowledge Communication.* 2018;1(1):515.

7. Yusoff, S. H. Western and Islamic Communication model: a comparative analysis on a theory application. *Journal of Islamic Social Sciences and Humanities.* 2016;7(1):7–20. http://dx.doi.org/10.12816/0029922

8. Azad, M. A. K. Principle of human communication: Islamic perspective. *RA Journal of Applied Research.* 2015;1 (6):227–31.

9. Fortner, R. S. & Fackler, P. M., eds. *The Handbook of Media and Mass Communication Theory.* Hoboken, NJ: Wiley-Blackwell. 2014.

10. Chouliaraki, L. Michel Foucault. In: Jensen, K. B. & Craig, T. R., eds. *International Encyclopedia of Communication Theory and Philosophy.* Hoboken, NJ: Wiley-Blackwell. 2016. https://doi.org/10.1002/9781118766804.wbiect236

11. Khalid, N. H. & Ahmad, F. A. Islamic-based art of communication framework. *International Journal of Academic Research in Business and Social Sciences.* 2021;11(7):24–34. http://dx.doi.org/10.6007/IJARBSS/v11-i7/10411

12. Thani, T., Idriss, I., Abubakar, M. A., & Idris, H. The teaching methods and techniques of the Prophet (PBUH): an exploratory study. *Journal Of Hadith Studies.* 2021;6(1):61–69. http://dx.doi.org/10.33102/johs.v6i1.128

13. Khan, I., Elius, M., Mohd Nor, M. R., Yakub Zulkifli, B. M., Noordin, K., & Mansor, F. A. A critical appraisal of interreligious dialogue in Islam. *SAGE Open.* 2020;10(4). https://doi.org/10.1177/2158244020970560

14. Ibrahim, H. Approaches to reading intercultural communication in the Qur'an and the politics of interpretation. *Critical Research on Religion.* 2014;2:99–115. https://doi.org/10.1177/2050303214535001

15. Khasanah, F. The Qur'anic communication ethics in social media: the significance of Surah Al-Hujurât. *Epistemé: Jurnal Pengembangan Ilmu Keislaman.* 2019;14(1):151–67. http://dx.doi.org/10.21274/epis.2019.14.1.151-167

16. Hossin, M. S., Ali, I., & Ilham, S. Human resource management practices from Islamic perspective: a study on Bangladesh context. *International Journal of Academic Research in Business and Social Sciences.* 2020;10(6):391–405. http://dx.doi.org/10.13140/RG.2.2.26073.54883

17. Ramlan, A. F., Suyurno, S., Sharipp, T., Ridzuan, A. R., Nur, S., & Faadiah, F. The influence of family communication in developing Muslim personality: an overview of family communication patterns theory. *E-Journal of Islamic Thought & Understanding.* 2019;1 (1):60–73.

18. Ghazizadeh, M. Islamic health sciences: a model for health education and promotion. *Journal of Health Education.* 1992;23(4):227–31. https://doi.org/10.1080/10556699.1992.10616296

19. Ghaly, M. Studies in Islamic ethics. In: Post, S. G., ed. *Encyclopedia of Bioethics.* 4th ed. New York: Macmillan Reference USA. 2018. 1–9.

20. Bayraklı, E. & Hafez, F. *Islamophobia in Muslim Majority Societies.* Milton Park, UK: Routledge. 2019.

21. Hashemi, N. *Islam, Secularism, and Liberal Democracy: Toward a Democratic Theory for Muslim Societies.* Oxford: Oxford University Press. 2012.

22. Al-Rasheed, M. *Muted Modernists: The Struggle Over Divine Politics in Saudi Arabia.* Oxford: Oxford University Press. 2016.

23. Hamada, B. Press freedom and political instability in the Arab world: an empirical investigation. *Journal of Arab & Muslim Media Research.* 2019;12:21–41. http://dx.doi.org/10.1386/jammr.12.1.21_1

24. Bianchi, R. R. *Islamic Globalization: Pilgrimage, Capitalism, Democracy, and Diplomacy.* 1st ed. Singapore: World Scientific Publishing Company. 2013.

25. Askari, H., Iqbal, Z., & Mirakhor, A. *Globalization and Islamic Finance: Convergence, Prospects, and Challenges.* Singapore: John Wiley & Sons (Asia) Pte. Ltd. 2010.

26. Hayder, S. A. Islam and social media entrepreneurial communications: the case of British Muslim entrepreneurs and their use of social media to identify markets and engage customers. Dissertation, Salford Business School, University of Salford, UK. 2018.

27. Bokhari, K. & Senzai, F. *Political Islam in the Age of Democratization.* London: Palgrave Macmillan. 2013.

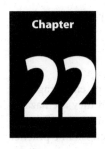

Contemporary Public Health, Islam, and Positive Health

Hassan Chamsi-Pasha, Mohammed Ali Albar

Introduction

Islam is a comprehensive way of life for all Muslims that covers personal, spiritual, social, financial, and political constructs. Muslims believe that religion cannot be separated from daily aspects of life. The Holy Qur'an and Prophetic guidance indicate that to live a content and productive life, one should have faith and put their faith into practice [1].

Islam emphasizes the significance of holistic well-being among individuals and communities. Numerous Qur'anic verses and traditions advocate health promoting activities. Spreading health mindfulness among Muslim physicians and patients using these verses is likely to have a strong effect on their attitudes [2].

This chapter explores the relationship between contemporary public health practices and the principles of Islam, highlighting the shared goals of promoting positive health and emphasizing the holistic approach to well-being promoted by Islamic teachings.

Religiosity and Health

Studies have explored the relationship between religiosity and health and its ability to prevent, treat, and facilitate successful coping with illness [3]. High levels of religiosity are associated with lower morbidity and mortality, enhanced quality of life and well-being, and lower incidence of depression and stress. Probable mechanisms include healthier lifestyle (e.g., healthy diets, smoking cessation, and alcohol abstention), lower rates of stress, and improvement of social ties [4]. A study in Norway revealed a significant correlation between Muslim religiosity and positive health outcomes, while there was no association between Muslim religiosity and negative health outcomes [5].

The Concept of Positive Health

In 2011, a contemporary conception of health was introduced. It was defined as the ability to adapt and to self-manage in the face of social, physical and emotional challenges [6]. This new conception was proposed because the traditional World Health Organization (WHO) description of health, which was defined as being in a state of complete physical, internal, and social well-being and not simply experiencing the absence of complaint or infirmity, was considered no longer acceptable [7]. The concept of positive health was developed to make this description measurable and includes six medical and nonmedical aspects: bodily functions, social participation, daily functioning, quality of life, meaningfulness, and mental well-being [7, 8]. Positive health focuses on the enablement of the patient by changing their lifestyle rather than just removing symptoms with medicine. People can perform their daily work and share in social activities and feel healthy despite constraints by successfully adapting to an illness [6].

Physical Health

Islam offers natural foundations of healthy living, and Muslims are encouraged to enhance their physical health. Islam prohibits religious practices when they are hazardous for the body. The Prophet Muhammad (PBUH) said, "A strong Muslim is better and is liked by Allah than a weak Muslim" [9]. A positive correlation between Islamic practice and better physical health is well established [5].

Lifestyle

The Qur'an provides divine wisdom towards a healthy life, and the lifestyle that the Qur'an inspires reduces the chances of people developing cardiovascular disease (CVD) by promoting healthy diet, physical exercise, engagement in spiritual activities, and abstention from prohibited foods and drinks [10]. According to the WHO, over 1 billion people worldwide are obese, including 340 million adolescents and 39 million children, and these numbers are steadily increasing. Obesity has been strongly associated with CVD, type 2 diabetes, hypertension, and cancer, and there is strong advocacy from the WHO for healthy lifestyle changes [11].

In the Qur'an, 28 verses were found concentrating on diet and nutrition, alcohol abstention, hygiene, and the significance of a healthy life. Drawing attention to these verses may serve as a health-promoting vehicle for public health physicians and health educators. Faith-based health promotion programs may make a strong impact on health behaviors within Muslim communities [12].

Islam has banned certain foods because of their ill-effects. The Qur'an states, "*O Believers! Eat of the good and pure things that we have provided for you*" (Q Al-Baqarah 2:172). Alcohol and gambling are also prohibited in Islam because of their negative effects on personal health and civic society. Most Islamic scholars prohibit smoking for its well-established deleterious effects [13]. Conversely, Islam stresses the importance of strengthening the body through physical activity [14].

Hygiene

The Prophet (PBUH) sanctioned the habit of washing hands before and after meals and said that "cleanliness is half faith" [15], putting great emphasis on the importance of always maintaining cleanliness [16]. Islam stresses washing private parts and hands after going to the toilet. 'Aisha, wife of the Prophet (PBUH), said, "I never saw the Messenger of Allah (PBUH) come out of the toilet without first (cleansing himself) with water" [17].

Fasting and Intermittent Fasting

In Islam, fasting involves abstaining from any drink or food between sunrise and sunset, whereas in intermittent fasting, calorie-free liquids such as water, coffee, and tea are allowed. For centuries, numerous Muslims have been performing voluntary fasting analogous to the intermittent fasting currently being advocated. 'Aisha recited, "The Prophet (PBUH) used to be keen to fast on Mondays and Thursday" [18]. Intermittent fasting has been shown to increase stress resistance, improve immune response, increase longevity, and reduce prevalence of chronic diseases [19, 20]. The effect of fasting on cardiovascular risk factors (e.g., blood glucose, lipid profile, and blood pressure) can be still seen during Ramadan fasting even without restricting caloric intake [21].

Social Health

Family Health

Family is often defined as the backbone of any society, and its structure affects the structure of the whole society. Despite the influence of modernization on many societies, several studies show religion as an outstanding factor in marriage and parenthood, and Islam honors the value of marriage as a legitimate response to the biological instinct for reproduction [22].

Intimate partner violence (IPV) is a major global health problem and a leading cause of homicide death for women. The WHO defines IPV as any behavior within an intimate relationship that leads to physical, psychological, or sexual harm to those in the relationship [23].

Approximately 30% of women worldwide experience some form of physical or sexual violence by an intimate partner during their life. Islamic values and principles support the protection of women from all forms of harm. The Islamic principles defend the status of women and consider them as full equal partners in the religious rights of Islam [24]. The Prophet (PBUH) instructed Muslims to protect and be kind to women: "The best of you is the one who is best to his wife" [25].

Sexual Health

The increase of sexual promiscuity plays a role in spreading sexually transmitted infections (STIs). Researchers estimate that on any given day one in five people in the United States have an STI [26]. Islam is strictly opposed to sexual relations outside of a defined legal marriage. This principle has a direct effect on reducing the incidence of STIs within Muslim communities [27].

Social Connections

Satisfaction with social relationships is considered a public health priority in the prevention of chronic diseases [28]. Poor social engagement with the elderly is associated with increased incidence of CVD, while good social engagement had positive effects on health outcomes [29]. Islam puts great emphasis on expressing kindness towards vulnerable groups such as the elderly, widows, orphans, and immigrants. Visiting the sick is encouraged in Islam and is considered a social support to the patient, which may be reflected in their positive health outcomes [30].

Financial Issues

Income inequality is a major factor that negatively affects health and well-being. Supporting the poor in Islam is corroborated through a) zakat, which obligates every able Muslim to pay alms to the poor, b) waqf, a charitable endowment frequently used in backing social development programs, and c) the prohibition of usury [30].

Daily Function

Islam fosters working, and the Prophet (PBUH) said, "Nobody has ever eaten a better meal than that which one has earned by working with one's own hands" [31]. Every day's activities that are routine in nature may convert to deeds if completed with the intentional purpose of worship. A recent meta-analysis revealed that sanctification of various aspects of life is associated with better positive psychosocial adjustment [32, 33].

Mental Health: An Islamic Holistic Perspective

Mental disorders are an increasing public health problem worldwide, and nearly 25% of adults and 10% of children may be affected by mental disorders annually with a substantial impact on the lives of millions of people [34]. Modern life that is associated with time pressure, social isolation, less sleep, and less connection with the family unit may predispose people to mental disorders, while religious practices and social connections have been shown to reduce and protect against depression and suicide [30].

Meaningfulness

Islam is a way of life and a set of guidelines for humans to achieve success in this world and the hereafter. This "way of life" requires Muslims to patiently face illness and hardships, and God will forgive their sins in response to their patience. The Prophet (PBUH) said, "Never a believer is stricken with a discomfort, an illness, an anxiety, a grief or mental worry, or even the pricking of a thorn, but Allah will expiate his sins on account of his patience" [35].

Quality of Life

The Prophet (PBUH) said, "Happy is the man who avoids dissension, but how fine is the man who is afflicted and shows endurance" [36]. The state of the peaceful self is reflected in the contentment with whatever God wishes (i.e., whatever happens in life). By adhering to the Islamic lifestyle, Muslims may experience positive emotions and pleasures (e.g., gratitude, contentment, vitality, peacefulness, joy etc.). The fundamental determinant of happiness and mental balance is the integration of these constructs via faith supplemented by a virtuous lifestyle [1]. Several studies have established a positive correlation between Muslim religiosity and satisfaction, higher subjective well-being, preventive health behavior, and mental health. A systematic review of 31 studies concluded that there was a positive association between Islamic faith and happiness [37].

Trusting God

The Prophet (PBUH) is cited as saying, "Say often, 'There is no strength nor power except God'" [38].

The Qur'an encourages Muslims to put their trust in God (*tawakkul*), as reflected in this verse: "*Put your trust in Allah: Allah is sufficient as Guardian*" (Q Al-Ahzaab 33:3). To Muslims, trusting God is essential in the face of distressing life events and when coping with hardship [33].

Non-Pharmacological Interventions

Anxiety is the most frequent mental disorder, and religion therapy has been indicated to be an effective intervention for anxiety management [34]. The traditional therapies utilize faith and trust in God, repentance, prayer, recitation of Qur'anic verses, and charity to the poor as healing factors since they are believed to reinforce the person's "soul" [1]. Remembrance of God is considered a soothing factor for Muslims: "*Verily in the remembrance of Allah do hearts find comfort*" (Q Ar-Ra'd 13:28).

Listening to the Holy Qur'an

Listening to the Qur'an has been indicated to serve as a form of spiritual-based therapy commonly used for addressing mental disorders. A systematic review demonstrated the positive effect of listening to the Qur'an in reducing anxiety [34]. Several verses in the Qur'an indicate its capability in healing and attaining tranquility: "*And We send down of the Qur'an that is healing and mercy for the believers*" (Q Al-Israa 17:82). Q Ar-Rahman was shown to reduce depression [39]. Listening to the Qur'an can be used as an adjunct to other established mental health treatments for Muslim patients.

Salat

In addition to the positive effects of salat on health including cardiovascular, neurological, and musculoskeletal effects, salat is believed to give spiritual nourishment and harmonize the emotional, spiritual, and mental aspects of the devotee and may be incorporated in rehabilitation programs and holistic care [4]. The Prophet (PBUH) said, "But my comfort has been handed in prayer" [40]. Studies have shown that salat resulted in the activation of the parasympathetic nervous system and a decrease in sympathetic activity [4]. A study of Muslim nurses showed a positive correlation between salat and life satisfaction and in reducing job stress [41]. Physicians may consider incorporating further mind–body techniques in view of the global increase in habitual stress-related disorders [42].

Conclusion

Islamic teachings of the Qur'an and Prophetic guidance can be viewed as a comprehensive spiritual, holistic, social, and mental guide governing all disciplines of a Muslim's life. Islam promotes healthy holistic lifestyle, promotes moderation, prohibits unhealthful habits, and inspires optimism and pliability in facing life's complexities. It upholds the sanctity of family life, promotes collective cooperation, and condemns conflicts and enmity.

References

1. Joshanloo, M. A comparison of Western and Islamic conceptions of happiness. *Journal of Happiness Studies.* 2013;14:1857–74. https://doi.org/10.1007/s10902-012-9406-7

2. Assad, S., Niazi, A. K., & Assad, S. Health and Islam. *Journal of Mid-Life Health.* 2013;4(1):65. https://doi.org/10.4103/0976-7800.109645

3. Al-Yousefi, N. A. Observations of Muslim physicians regarding the influence of religion on health and their clinical approach. *Journal of Religion and Health.* 2012;51(2):269–80. https://doi.org/10.1007/s10943-012-9567-z

4. Chamsi-Pasha, M. & Chamsi-Pasha, H. A review of the literature on the health benefits of salat (Islamic prayer). *The Medical Journal of Malaysia.* 2021;76(1):93–97.

5. Ishaq, B., Østby, L., & Johannessen, A. Muslim religiosity and health outcomes: a cross-sectional study among Muslims in Norway. *SSM Population Health.* 2021;15

(100843):1–7. https://doi.org/10.1016/j
.ssmph.2021.100843

6. Huber, M., Knottnerus, J. A., Green, L., van der Horst, H., Jadad, A. R., Kromhout, D., et al. How should we define health? *The BMJ*. 2011;343:d4163. https://doi.org/10.1136/bmj.d4163

7. Huber, M., van Vliet, M., Giezenberg, M., Winkens, B., Heerkens, Y., Dagnelie, P. C., et al. Towards a "patient-centred" operationalisation of the new dynamic concept of health: a mixed methods study. *BMJ Open*. 2016;6(1): e010091. https://doi.org/10.1136/bmjopen-2015-010091

8. Bodryzlova, Y. & Moullec, G. Definitions of positive health: a systematic scoping review. *Global Health Promotion*. 2023;30 (3):6–14. https://doi.org/10.1177/17579759221139802

9. Sahih Muslim. *Sahih Muslim 2664*. In-book reference: Book 46, Hadith 52. Available from: https://sunnah.com/muslim:2664

10. Turgut, O., Yalta, K., & Tandogan, I. Islamic legacy of cardiology: inspirations from the holy sources. *International Journal of Cardiology*. 2010;145(3):496. https://doi.org/10.1016/j.ijcard.2009.09.470

11. Aboul-Enein, B. H. "The Qur'anic garden": consumption of fruits, vegetables, and whole grains from an Islamic perspective. *International Journal of Multicultural and Multireligious Understanding*. 2017;4(4):53–63. http://dx.doi.org/10.18415/ijmmu.v4i4.78

12. Aboul-Enein, B. H. Health-promoting verses as mentioned in the Holy Qur'an. *Journal of Religion and Health*. 2016;55 (3):821–29. https://doi.org/10.1007/s10943-014-9857-8

13. Ghouri, N., Atcha, M., & Sheikh, A. Influence of Islam on smoking among Muslims. *The BMJ*. 2006;332 (7536):291–94. https://doi.org/10.1136/bmj.332.7536.291

14. Chamsi-Pasha, H. Islam and the cardiovascular patient: pragmatism in practice. *The British Journal of Cardiology*. 2013;20(3):1–4. http://dx.doi.org/10.5837/bjc.2013.020

15. Sahih Muslim. *Sahih Muslim 223*. In-book reference: Book 2, Hadith 1. Available from: https://sunnah.com/muslim:223

16. Chamsi-Pasha, H. & Mousa, S. A. Healthy living and lifestyle with Prophet teaching. *Journal of Agricultural Safety and Health*. 2021;2(1):1–10.

17. Sunan Ibn Majah. *Sunan Ibn Majah 354*. In-book reference: Book 1, Hadith 88. Available from: https://sunnah.com/ibnmajah:354

18. Sunan an-Nasa'i. *Sunan an-Nasa'i 2364*. In-book reference: Book 22, Hadith 275. Available from: https://sunnah.com/nasai:2364

19. de Cabo, R. & Mattson, M. P. Effects of intermittent fasting on health, aging, and disease. *The New England Journal of Medicine*. 2019;381 (26):2541–51. https://doi.org/10.1056/nejmra1905136

20. Ealey, K. N., Phillips, J., & Sung, H. K. COVID-19 and obesity: fighting two pandemics with intermittent fasting. *Trends in Endocrinology & Metabolism*. 2021;32(9):706–20. https://doi.org/10.1016/j.tem.2021.06.004

21. Dong, T. A., Sandesara, P. B., Dhindsa, D. S., Mehta, A., Arneson, L. C., Dollar, A. L., et al. Intermittent fasting: a heart healthy dietary pattern? *The American Journal of Medicine*. 2020;133(8):901–7. https://doi.org/10.1016/j.amjmed.2020.03.030

22. Abd Rahman, A. & Mahmud, A. A review of the Islamic approach in public health practices. *International Journal of Public Health and Clinical Sciences*. 2014;1 (2):1–14.

23. World Health Organization. *Understanding and Addressing Violence against Women*. 2012. Available from: https://apps.who.int/iris/bitstream/handle/10665/77432/WHO_RHR_12.36_eng.pdf

24. Chamsi-Pasha, H., Chamsi-Pasha, M., & Albar, M. A. Violence against women during COVID-19 pandemic restrictions. *The BMJ*. 2020;369:m1712. https://doi.org/10.1136/bmj.m1712

25. Sunan Ibn Majah. *Sunan Ibn Majah 1977.* In-book reference: Book 9, Hadith 133. Available from: https://sunnah.com/ ibnmajah:1977

26. Center for Disease Control and Prevention. CDC estimates 1 in 5 people in the U.S. have a sexually transmitted infection. [online]. 2021 [Accessed December 15, 2022]. Available from: https://archive.cdc.gov/#/details? url=https://www.cdc.gov/media/releases/ 2021/p0125-sexualy-transmitted-infection.html

27. El-Hamdoon, O. H. Islam and public health. *Journal of the British Islamic Medical Association.* 2021;8(3):50–53.

28. Xu, X., Mishra, G. D., Holt-Lunstad, J., & Jones, M. Social relationship satisfaction and accumulation of chronic conditions and multimorbidity: a national cohort of Australian women. *General Psychiatry.* 2023;36(1):e100925. https://doi.org/10 .1136/gpsych-2022-100925

29. Coyte, A., Perry, R., Papacosta, A. O., Lennon, L., Whincup, P. H., Wannamethee, S. G., et al. Social relationships and the risk of incident heart failure: results from a prospective population-based study of older men. *European Heart Journal Open.* 2021;2(1): oeab045. https://doi.org/10.1093/ ehjopen/oeab045

30. Yunus, R. M. Public health: an Islamic perspective. *International Journal of Islamic Thoughts.* 2017;6(2):69–82.

31. Sahih al-Bukhari. *Sahih al-Bukhari 2072.* In-book reference: Book 34, Hadith 25. Available from: https://sunnah.com/ bukhari:2072

32. Mahoney, A., Wong, S., Pomerleau, J. M., & Pargament, K. I. Sanctification of diverse aspects of life and psychosocial functioning: a meta-analysis of studies from 1999 to 2019. *Psychology of Religion and Spirituality.* 2022;14(4):585–98. https://doi.org/10.1037/rel0000354

33. Saritoprak, S. M. & Abu-Raiya, H. Living the good life: an Islamic perspective on positive psychology. In: Davis, E. B., Worthington, E. L., Jr., & Schnitker, S. A., eds. *Handbook of Positive Psychology,*

Religion and Spirituality. Cham, CH: Springer. 2023. 179–93.

34. Abd-alrazaq, A., Malkawi, A. A., Maabreh, A. H., Alam, T., Bewick, B. M., Akhu-Zaheya, L., et al. The effectiveness of listening to the Holy Qur'an to improve mental disorders and psychological wellbeing: Systematic review and meta-analysis. [preprint]. *Research Square.* 2020:1–25. https://doi .org/10.21203/rs.3.rs-44376/v1

35. Sahih Muslim. *Sahih Muslim 2573.* In-book reference: Book 45, Hadith 66. Available from: https://sunnah.com/muslim:2573

36. Sunan Abi Dawud. *Sunan Abi Dawud 4263.* In-book reference: Book 37, Hadith 24. Available from: https://sunnah.com/ abudawud:4263

37. Rizvi, M. A. K. & Hossain, M. Z. Relationship between religious belief and happiness: a systematic literature review. *Journal of Religion and Health.* 2017;56 (5):1561–82. https://doi.org/10.1007/ s10943-016-0332-6

38. Sahih al-Bukhari. *Sahih al-Bukhari 613.* In-book reference: Book 10, Hadith 11. Available from: https://sunnah.com/ bukhari:613

39. Rafique, R., Anjum, A., & Raheem, S. S. Efficacy of Surah Al-Rehman in managing depression in Muslim women. *Journal of Religion and Health.* 2019;58 (2):516–26. https://doi.org/10.1007/ s10943-017-0492-z

40. Sunan an-Nasa'i. *Sunan an-Nasa'i 3939.* In-book reference: Book 36, Hadith 1. Available from: https://sunnah.com/ nasai:3939

41. Achour, M., Muhamad, A., Syihab, A. H., Mohd Nor, M. R., & Mohd Yusoff, M. Y. Z. Prayer moderating job stress among Muslim nursing staff at the University of Malaya Medical Centre (UMMC). *Journal of Religion and Health.* 2019;60 (1):202–20. https://doi.org/10.1007/ s10943-019-00834-6

42. Saniotis, A. Understanding mind/body medicine from Muslim religious practices of salat and dhikr. *Journal of Religion and Health.* 2018;57(3):849–57. https://doi .org/10.1007/s10943-014-9992-2

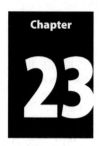

Chapter 23

Cultural Competence in Public Health: A Brief Islamic Perspective

Noura Mostafa Mohamed, Fatmah Almoayad,
Nada Benajiba

Introduction

This chapter introduces professional cultural competence in public health with its relation to Islam. This is a brief overview of the concept of cultural competency and its significance in health care from an Islamic perspective. This chapter also emphasizes the contemporary challenges faced by public health professionals in understanding their community's religious and spiritual beliefs when making medical and health decisions.

Cultural Competence

Cultural competence encompasses a comprehensive blend of behaviors, attitudes, and policies among professionals facilitating work in a diverse cultural context [1]. Specifically, "culture" refers to the integrated patterns of human behavior that include language, thoughts, communications, actions, customs, beliefs, values, and institutions of racial, ethnic, religious, or social groups. While cultural competence signifies the ability of both individuals and organizations to operate proficiently within different cultural frameworks, cultural incompetence may lead to patients receiving poor quality care, leading to negative health consequences and poor health outcomes [2].

Cultural Competence from an Islamic Perspective

Though Islamic texts do not directly reference cultural competence, they do highlight fundamental principles that align with its values and concepts. Derived from the Holy Qur'an and Sunnah, these principles, such as *Ihsan* (excellence), *Ta'awun* (cooperation), honest work earning, *Karamah* (dignity), *Adel* (justice), fulfilling responsibilities, and *Shura* (consultation), underscore the importance of understanding and respecting diverse cultures [3]. In addition to these principles, there is also the principle known as *Kafa'ah*, which is regarded as expertise and skills in the areas of work performed. Given that health care professionals should be qualified and competent to perform their tasks, Islam cautions against entrusting responsibilities to individuals who lack expertise, as doing so is seen as a betrayal to God (Allah), His Messenger Muhammad (PBUH), and the community.

One of the requirements of achieving competency in work is acknowledging that helping people is regarded as a form of worship to Allah. The more the health professional becomes proficient in their work towards people using competent practices, the more the health care provider will strengthen their position in the community and their health care settings [4]. The Holy Qur'an states, "*O ye who believe! If ye will aid (the cause of) Allah, He will assist you, and plant your feet firmly*" (Q Muhammad 47:7).

Noteworthy also is the verse of the Holy Qur'an Q An-Nahl 16:90, which states, "*Indeed, Allah orders justice and good conduct and giving to relatives and forbids immorality and bad conduct and oppression. He admonishes you that perhaps you will be reminded.*"

Another requirement of competencies is *Amanah*, which has the same root as *Amin* and means "honesty, trustworthiness, and integrity." One with the title *Al-Amin*, meaning "the trusted one," is regarded as a person who is trusted and competent if given a task to perform or shows *Amanah* towards them because they will take responsibility for the task appointed to them. Using *Amanah*, people will feel secure from betrayal, cheating, lying, and breaking promises [5].

Cultural Competence in Muslim Communities

Cultural competence is imperative when addressing health disparities and ensuring quality health care delivery among diverse populations, including Muslims. A nuanced understanding of Islamic beliefs, practices, and cultural norms is crucial in fostering a health care environment that is both respectful and responsive to the unique needs of Muslim patients. A systematic review of 53 studies across a wide range of countries indicates a consistent relationship between experiences of discrimination, Islamophobia, and adverse health outcomes among Muslim populations [6]. Discrimination, particularly due to Muslim identity, showed consistent correlations with worsened mental health states such as psychological distress and depressive symptoms [7, 8]. Hence, public health should consider cultural competence as a key in mitigating the impacts of discrimination and Islamophobia. This can facilitate open and empathetic communication, ensuring that the health care needs of Muslim patients are met with sensitivity and without bias or prejudice. Such an approach promotes trust, encourages health care-seeking behaviors, and contributes to more effective and equitable health care services, addressing the broader determinants of health and well-being in Muslim communities. In doing so, cultural competence acts as a buffer against the negative repercussions of discrimination, enhancing the overall health outcomes of Muslim patients [6].

Cultural Competence in the Care of a Muslim Patient

The provisions of health care need to include the cultural, religious, and spiritual needs of the respective patient. Thus, health care professionals should be empowered with the knowledge and skills to respond and pay special attention to the needs of patients and their families [9].

Religion and spirituality are critical factors that comprise the health-related constructs involved in patients seeking care. Health care providers who lack cultural competence training often neglect or omit taking religious beliefs into account when making medical decisions or offering guidance to patients and their families [10]. One of the challenges facing public health practitioners and health professionals is acknowledging that patients often consult their spiritual leaders and religious doctrines when making health-related decisions and seeking health advice [11]. In fact, it is demonstrated that religion and spirituality can affect decisions on dietary patterns, medications, and the preferred sex of their health providers [12].

Islam has strict prayer times and fasting periods that may interfere with medical treatment, health education, and administration [13]. Because of this, health care professionals should recognize and accommodate the patient's religious and spiritual requirements. As such, public health practitioners should grant an opportunity for Muslims to discuss their religious and spiritual beliefs and tailor their evaluation and treatment to meet their specific needs and demands [9].

Clinical Consideration When Looking after Muslim Patients

Many Muslims believe that good health involves the intertwining of physical, psychological, spiritual, and social factors. Good health is considered a blessing that God has given humankind. Muslim patients often respond to illness with patience, prayers, and meditation. In terms of dietary intake and drug administration, Ramadan fasting could cause a common experience where fasting Muslims create a challenge for the administration of drugs as they may refuse treatment [14, 15].

Health care professionals need to take the time to explain the importance of a medication to the patient and demonstrate flexibility and adaptation in the best interest of the patient. Hence, an informed and respectful approach will help the patient make the most culturally congruent decision depending on the health condition and treatment administration [16]. Another aspect of consideration among Muslim patients is their emphasis on privacy. Muslims tend to prefer to receive their medical care from a health care professional of the same sex. This is particularly crucial if the patient requires sex-specific care, such as obstetric/gynecologic or urologic care. If sex-specific care is not feasible, particularly for female patients, a female staff member or relative of the patient should be present during examinations and health communication [13, 17].

Some Muslims use traditional remedies based on the Holy Qur'an, Hadith, and Sunnah of the Prophet Muhammad (PBUH) [13, 18]. These treatments may include the use or consumption of aloe, dates, dill, fenugreek, pomegranate, or olives [13, 19]. Most of these are likely to be harmless, but some may be unsafe in the case of excessive use. Consequently, health care providers are encouraged to inquire with regards to the use of complementary or alternative treatment the Muslim patient might be using, particularly as it relates to potential drug interactions.

Health care professionals should familiarize themselves with the practices and procedures of worship and Islamic prayer, such as the requirement of ablution and the necessity to face the direction of Mecca during prayer, known as the *Qibla*. Whenever possible, health care professionals should assist Muslim patients in determining the direction to Mecca. In addition, once prayer begins, the health care provider should be respectful of giving the patient privacy and a place to pray and avoid all kinds of interruptions as the prayer commences. Bedridden patients may choose to pray in bed or in a chair, and disability-supportive assistance should be accessible [20].

Conclusion

The fundamentals of cultural competencies are inherently part of Islamic values and can be applied universally across all health care settings. Islamic beliefs affect Muslim patients' attitudes, beliefs, and behavior. Thus, Muslims perceive the doctrines of Islam as a religion that provides instructions and guidelines that encompass a Muslim's life, where different aspects of life are integrated including health care and treatment. By understanding this, it becomes clear that the care of Muslim patients requires meeting the specific needs of religious practices and procedures whenever present. Additionally, to address the prevalent issue of Islamophobia and discrimination, health care professionals should intensify their efforts in reflecting upon these cultural congruencies. This will enhance their ability to navigate the challenges Muslim patients and communities face, ensuring the provision of culturally sensitive and respectful care.

References

1. Cross, T., Bazron, B., Dennis, K., & Isaacs, M. *Towards a Culturally Competent System of Care.* Vol. 1. Washington, DC: Georgetown University Child Development Center, CASSP Technical Assistance Center. 1989.

2. Fleckman, J. M., Dal Corso, M., Ramirez, S., Begalieva, M., & Johnson, C. C. Intercultural competency in public health: a call for action to incorporate training into public health education. *Frontiers in Public Health.* 2015;3:210. https://doi.org/10.3389/fpubh.2015.00210

3. Al Smadi, A. N., Amaran, S., Arriff, T. M., & Alown, B. Development and validation of a new Islamic work ethics scale for healthcare providers in emergency departments (EDIWES). *Journal of Islamic Business and Management.* 2021;11(2):312–27.

4. Batalden, P., Leach, D., Swing, S., Dreyfus, H., & Dreyfus, S.. General competencies and accreditation in graduate medical education. *Health Affairs.* 2002;21(5):103–11. https://doi.org/10.1377/hlthaff.21.5.103

5. Riyad as-Salihin. *Riyad as-Salihin 199.* In-book reference: Introduction, Hadith 199. Available from: https://sunnah.com/riyadussalihin:199

6. Samari, G., Alcalá, H. E., & Sharif, M. Z. Islamophobia, health, and public health: a systematic literature review. *American Journal of Public Health.* 2018;108(6): e1–9. https://doi.org/10.2105/AJPH.2018.304402

7. Abdulrahim, S., James, S. A., Yamout, R., & Baker, W. Discrimination and psychological distress: does whiteness matter for Arab Americans? *Social Science & Medicine.* 2012;75(12):2116–23. https://doi.org/10.1016/j.socscimed.2012.07.030

8. Aprahamian, M., Kaplan, D. M., Windham, A. M., Sutter, J. A., & Visser, J. The relationship between acculturation and mental health of Arab Americans. *Journal of Mental Health Counseling.* 2011;33(1):80–92. https://doi.org/10.17744/mehc.33.1.0356488305383630

9. Swihart, D. L., Yarrarapu, S. N. S., & Martin, R. L. *Cultural Religious Competence in Clinical Practice.* In: StatPearls [online]. Treasure Island, FL: StatPearls Publishing. 2022. Available from: www.ncbi.nlm.nih.gov/books/NBK493216/

10. Abdel-Razig, S., Ibrahim, H., Alameri, H., Hamdy, H., Haleeqa, K. A., Qayed, K. I., et al. Creating a framework for medical professionalism: an initial consensus statement from an Arab nation. *Journal of Graduate Medical Education.* 2016;8 (2):165–72. https://doi.org/10.4300/jgme-d-15-00310.1

11. Epner, D. E. & Baile, W. F. Patient-centered care: the key to cultural competence. *Annals of Oncology.* 2012;23 (Suppl 3):33–42. https://doi.org/10.1093/annonc/mds086

12. LeDoux, J., Mann, C., Demoratz, M., & Young, J. Addressing spiritual and religious influences in care delivery. *Professional Case Management.* 2019;24 (3):142–47. https://doi.org/10.1097/ncm.0000000000000346

13. Attum, B., Hafiz, S., Malik, A., & Shamoon, Z. *Cultural Competence in the Care of Muslim Patients and Their Families.* In: StatPearls [online]. Treasure Island, FL: StatPearls Publishing. 2023. Available from: www.ncbi.nlm.nih.gov/books/NBK499933/

14. éMutair, A. S., Plummer, V., O'Brien, A. P., & Clerehan, R. Providing culturally congruent care for Saudi patients and their families. *Contemporary Nurse.*

2014;46(2):254–58. https://doi.org/10.5172/conu.2014.46.2.254

15. Amin, M. E. K. & Abdelmageed, A. Clinicians' perspectives on caring for Muslim patients considering fasting during Ramadan. *Journal of Religion and Health.* 2020;59(3):1370–87. https://doi.org/10.1007/s10943-019-00820-y

16. Chehovich, C., Demler, T. L., & Leppien, E. Impact of Ramadan fasting on medical and psychiatric health. *International Clinical Psychopharmacology.* 2019;34(6):317–22. https://doi.org/10.1097/yic.0000000000000275

17. Douki, S., Ben Zineb, S., Nacef, F., & Halbreich, U. Women's mental health in the Muslim world: cultural, religious, and social issues. *Journal of Affective Disorders.* 2007;102(1–3):177–89. https://doi.org/10.1016/j.jad.2006.09.027

18. Blankinship, L. A. Providing culturally sensitive care for Islamic patients and families. *Journal of Christian Nursing.* 2018;35(2):94–99. https://doi.org/10.1097/cnj.0000000000000418

19. Rassool, G. H. *Cultural Competence in Caring for Muslim Patients.* Basingstoke, UK: Palgrave Macmillan. 2014.

20. Ding, M., Johnston, A. N. B., Mohammed, O. A., Luong, K., & Massey, D. Do consumers who identify as Muslim experience culturally safe care (CSC) in the emergency department (ED)? A scoping review. *Australasian Emergency Care.* 2018;21(3):93–98. https://doi.org/10.1016/j.auec.2018.08.001

Chapter 24

Muslims and Non-Muslims: Perspectives on Immigrant and Minority Health

Elizabeth Dodge

Introduction

Health practices and principles are influenced by many factors, including religious beliefs [1-4]. Additionally, social determinants of health, including built environments, socioeconomic status and economic stability, access to and quality of education and health care, and social and community resourcing and relationships, can all contribute to health practices, beliefs, and outcomes [5-8]. In Muslim Majority Countries (MMCs), Islamic principles can inform public health practice, approaches to nutrition, and health care [9, 10, 11], but given the presence of many non-Muslims in these societies, including patients and caregivers, adequate understanding and appropriate application of these principles is necessary to achieve the best public and individual health outcomes for all.

Health Outcomes in Muslim Majority Countries and Communities

There is a paucity in the literature that explores the health care and public health experiences of non-Muslim populations in MMCs [12, 13]. However, there is a growing body of research devoted to non-Muslim and expatriate caregivers both in MMCs and in countries and communities where there are large Muslim populations. A comprehensive study of health indicators (life expectancy, maternal mortality ratio, and infant mortality rate) and disparities in MMCs found worse national health indicators and health outcomes in MMCs compared to non-MMCs with four main predictive determinants: gross national income, literacy rate, access to clean water, and the corruption prediction index [14]. A comparative analysis of maternal and child health in the Islamic world found that while there have been improvements in some health indicators based on the Sustainable Development Goals, MMCs had higher mortality rates compared globally with other countries, and they had variation among other health indicators based on individual countries' structural and contextual determinants [8].

Factors that affect health outcomes in MMCs (such as reproductive health, pre- and postnatal care including labor and delivery, and childhood vaccination status) include refugee populations, political stability (or the absence thereof), political rights, government effectiveness, gross national income, total literacy, and female literacy [8]. In relation to vaccination hesitancy and potential caution regarding pharmaceuticals, it is important for care providers to understand and offer options for *halal* medicines and pharmaceutical components and for them to be able to provide this information to Muslim patients [15]. Regarding some of the other identified determinants related to health outcomes, a review of culture and language differences among expatriate and non-

Muslim health care workers in Saudi Arabia found that language barriers and the lack of cultural knowledge about Muslim practices such as breastfeeding, food restrictions, and modesty caused issues including errors in treatment, perceived poor quality care, and, in some instances, was attributed to the cause of death in Muslim patients seeking care [16]. Amid a shortage of Saudi nurses (in the Saudi Arabian nursing workforce, expatriate nurses constitute 63.82%, while only 32.3% of nurses are Saudi nurses), researchers found a significant positive correlation between the cultural competence of expatriate and non-Muslim nurses and patient perception of the provision of patient-centered care [17].

Cultural Humility, Health, and Immigrant Populations

Cultural humility, or competency, in public health and health workers is a critical skill affecting public health and health outcomes in countries and communities with immigrant Muslim populations when compared to non-Muslim peers [17, 18, 19]. While Muslim immigrants are at increased risk for diabetes and some cancers and may need to seek mental health care [20–23], they may choose to forego recommended screenings, miss appointments, and not understand or agree to plans of care when such plans are not aligned with their cultural and religious beliefs. Therefore, health care workers and public health partners should educate practitioners on culturally relevant care practices and consult local communities on how to inform best practice in accordance with their belief systems [8, 24, 25]. Parallel to the implementation and integration of culturally relevant care, which should be available to all patients regardless of belief systems, Islamophobia should be addressed as a barrier to immigrant Muslim populations accessing health care services. Studies have noted that Islamophobia, on the rise in Europe and the US and compounded by the 2017 "Muslim ban" [26] (repealed in 2021 [27]), has adversely affected health care in the Muslim population in the US [7, 28]. Health care providers must understand and address the barriers to equitable health care access and approach these with cultural humility.

Culturally Congruent Public Health Promotion

In addition to primary health care settings, it is important to understand how to implement initiatives in support of public health for Muslim communities, specifically where culturally sensitive nuances exist, such as with sex education, tobacco use, vaccination hesitancy, and domestic violence [29–32]. When public health partners work collaboratively with the community or communities intended to benefit from an initiative, the initiative is more likely to be successful [24, 25]. Another important determinant of public health and health outcomes is access to culturally congruent foods in both MMCs and non-MMCs with a Muslim population. Logistical and monetary disincentives posed in the procurement and transport of *halal* foods even in MMCs is a barrier to *halal* food supply chains [33, 34]. However, research proposes several approaches to increasing non-Muslim understanding and acceptance/purchasing of *halal* foods that may help remove these barriers, such as educating non-Muslims on the health benefits of *halal* food, highlighting the animal welfare considerations of *halal* food production, processing, and manufacturing, and relying on Muslim friends and family to inform non-Muslims on brands they enjoy, thereby increasing brand recognition [33–37]. There is growing interest in and adoption of *halal* food purchasing by non-Muslims in MMCs. Non-Muslim consumers can be encouraged to view *halal* food as an accessible and healthy option to include in their diets. Accordingly, producers and transporters will continue to invest where there is interest, helping to surmount the barrier of financing transportation and distribution of *halal* foods.

Conclusion

Based on the examination of non-Muslims in Muslim societies, there is a paucity in the literature about the public health and health outcomes of non-Muslim minorities in MMCs. Cultural humility, education in cultural competence, and a reliance on collaborative work within communities to attain positive public health and health outcomes is of utmost importance regardless of faith. In MMCs that are disproportionality impacted by war, government corruption, low literacy rates, low national income, and limited access to clean water, it is critical that Muslim and non-Muslim health care practitioners, public health partners, and other stakeholders work together towards changes that support the health outcomes of the society as a whole. Non-Muslims, both in health care and public health professions as well as those residing in MMCs or societies with a large Muslim population, can work to cultivate an understanding of how Muslim religious beliefs and values intersect with a variety of public health topics, health care, and foodways. Through a mutual understanding of how these factors relate to and interface with the social determinants of health and through collective action to improve these areas, all community members can be supported in achieving better public health and health care outcomes.

References

1. Johnson, K. S., Elbert-Avila, K. I., & Tulsky, J. A. The influence of spiritual beliefs and practices on the treatment preferences of African Americans: a review of the literature. *Journal of the American Geriatrics Society*. 2005;53(4) 711–19. https://doi.org/10.1111/j.1532-5415.2005.53224.x

2. Hag Hamed, D. & Daniel, M. The influence of fatalistic beliefs on health beliefs among diabetics in Khartoum, Sudan: a comparison between Coptic Christians and Sunni Muslims. *Global Health Promotion*. 2019;26(3):15–22. https://doi.org/10.1177/1757975917715884

3. Musa, A. S., Pevalin, D. J., & Shahin, F. I. Impact of spiritual well-being, spiritual perspective, and religiosity on the self-rated health of Jordanian Arab Christians. *Journal of Transcultural Nursing*. 2016;27

(6):550–57. https://doi.org/10.1177/1043659615587590

4. Tackett, S., Young, J. H., Putman, S., Wiener, C., Deruggiero, K., & Bayram, J. D. Barriers to healthcare among Muslim women: a narrative review of the literature. *Women's Studies International Forum*. 2018;69:190–94. https://doi.org/10.1016/j.wsif.2018.02.009

5. OASH. Social determinants of health. [online]. Healthy People 2030. 2023 [Accessed May 17, 2023]. Available from: https://health.gov/healthypeople/priority-areas/social-determinants-health

6. World Health Organization. Social determinants of health. [online]. 2023 [Accessed May 17, 2023]. Available from: www.who.int/health-topics/social-determinants-of-health#tab=tab_1

7. Samari, G., Alcalá, H. E., & Sharif, M. Z. Islamophobia, health, and public health: a systematic literature review. *American Journal of Public Health*. 2018;108(6):

e1–e9. https://doi.org/10.2105/AJPH.2018
.304402

8. Akseer, N., Kamali, M., Bakhache, N.,
Mirza, M., Mehta, S., Al-Gashm, S., et al.
Status and drivers of maternal, newborn,
child and adolescent health in the Islamic
world: a comparative analysis. *The Lancet.*
2018;391(10129):1493–512. https://doi
.org/10.1016/s0140-6736(18)30183-1

9. Khalid, S. M. N. & Sediqi, S. M.
Improving nutritional and food security
status in Muslim communities:
integration of Qur'anic practices in
development programs – a review.
*International Journal of Nutrition
Sciences.* 2018;3(2):65–72.

10. Hibban, M. F. Living Qur'an and Sunnah
as the foundation of a holistic healthy
lifestyle. *International Journal of Islamic
and Complementary Medicine.* 2022;3
(2):49–56. https://doi.org/10.55116/
IJICM.V3I2.40

11. Rassool, H. G. Cultural competence in
nursing Muslim patients. *Nursing Times.*
2015;111(14):12–15.

12. Bansal, B., Takkar, J., Soni, N. D.,
Agrawal, D. K., & Agarwal, S.
Comparative study of prevalence of
anemia in Muslim and non-Muslim
pregnant women of western Rajasthan.
*International Journal of Research in
Health Sciences.* 2013;1(2):47–52.

13. Hanif, A. A., Hasan, M., Khan, M. S.,
Hossain, M. M., Shamim, A. A.,
Hossaine, M., et al. Ten-years
cardiovascular risk among Bangladeshi
population using non-laboratory-based
risk chart of the World Health
Organization: findings from a nationally
representative survey. *PLoS ONE.* 2021;16
(5):e0251967. https://doi.org/10.1371/
journal.pone.0251967

14. Razzak, J. A., Khan, U. R., Azam, I.,
Nasrullah, M., Pasha, O., Malik M., et al.
Health disparities between Muslim and
non-Muslim countries. *EMHJ: Eastern
Mediterranean Health Journal.* 2011;17
(9):654–64.

15. Khan, T. M. & Shaharuddin, S. Need for
contents on *halal* medicines in pharmacy

and medicine curriculum. *Archives of
Pharmacy Practice.* 2015;6(2):38–40.

16. Almutairi, K. M. Culture and language
differences as a barrier to provision of
quality care by the health workforce in
Saudi Arabia. *Saudi Medical Journal.*
2015;36(4):425–31. https://doi.org/10
.15537/smj.2015.4.10133

17. Albougami, A. S., Alotaibi, J. S.,
Alsharari, A. F., Albagawi, B. S., Almazan,
J. U., Maniago, J. D., et al. Cultural
competence and perception of patient-
centered care among non-Muslim
expatriate nurses in Saudi Arabia: a cross
sectional study. *Pakistan Journal of
Medical & Health Sciences.* 2019;13
(2):933–39.

18. Yosef, A. R. Health beliefs, practice, and
priorities for health care of Arab Muslims
in the United States. *Journal of
Transcultural Nursing.* 2008;19
(3):284–91. https://doi.org/10.1177/
1043659608317450

19. Ezenkwele, U. A. & Roodsari, G. S.
Cultural competencies in emergency
medicine: caring for Muslim-American
patients from the Middle East. *The
Journal of Emergency Medicine.* 2013;45
(2):168–74. https://doi.org/10.1016/j
.jemermed.2012.11.077

20. Jaber, L., Brown, M., Hammad, A., Zhu,
Q., & Herman, W. Lack of acculturation
is a risk factor for diabetes in Arab
immigrants in the US. *Diabetes Care.*
2003;26(7):2010–14. https://doi.org/10
.2337/diacare.26.7.2010

21. Kazi, E., Sareshwala, S., Ansari, Z.,
Sahota, D., Katyal, T., Tseng, W., et al.
Promoting colorectal cancer screening in
South Asian Muslims living in the USA.
Journal of Cancer Education. 2021;36
(4):865–73. https://doi.org/10.1007/
s13187-020-01715-3

22. Racine, L., D'Souza, M. S., & Tinampay,
C. Effectiveness of breast cancer screening
interventions in improving screening
rates and preventive activities in Muslim
refugee and immigrant women: a
systematic review and meta-analysis.
Journal of Nursing Scholarship. 2023;55

(1):329–44. https://doi.org/10.1111/jnu
.12818

23. Bagasra, A. Religious interpretations of
mental illness and help-seeking
experiences among Muslim Americans:
implications for clinical practice.
Spirituality in Clinical Practice. 2023;10
(1):20–31. https://doi.org/10.1037/
scp0000299

24. Heirali, A. A., Javed, S., Damani, Z.,
Kachra, R., Valiani, S., Walli, A. K., et al.
Muslim perspectives on advance care
planning: a model for community
engagement. *Palliative Care & Social
Practice.* 2021;15:1–6. https://doi.org/10
.1177/2632352421997152

25. Abu-Ras, W. & Laird, L. How Muslim
and non-Muslim chaplains serve Muslim
patients? Does the interfaith chaplaincy
model have room for Muslims'
experiences? *Journal of Religion and
Health.* 2011;50:46–61. https://doi.org/10
.1007/s10943-010-9357-4

26. Department of Homeland Security,
Department of Justice. *Executive Order
Protecting The Nation From Foreign
Terrorist Entry Into The United States.*
2018. Available from: www.dhs.gov/
sites/default/files/publications/
Executive%20Order%2013780%
20Section%2011%20Report%20-%
20Final.pdf

27. Biden, J. R., Jr. Proclamation on ending
discriminatory bans on entry to the
United States. [online]. The White
House. 2021 [Accessed June 7, 2023].
Available from: www.whitehouse.gov/
briefing-room/presidential-actions/
2021/01/20/proclamation-ending-
discriminatory-bans-on-entry-to-the-
united-states/

28. Samuels, E. A., Orr, L., White, E. B.,
Saadi, A., Padela, A. I., Westerhaus, M.,
et al. Health care utilization before and
after the "Muslim Ban" executive order
among people born in Muslim-majority
countries and living in the US. *JAMA
Network Open.* 2021;4(7):e2118216.
https://doi.org/10.1001/jamanetworkopen
.2021.18216

29. Smerecnik, C., Schaalma, H., Gerjo, K.,
Meijer, S., & Poelman, J. An exploratory
study of Muslim adolescents' views on
sexuality: implications for sex education
and prevention. *BMC Public Health.*
2010;10:1–10. https://doi.org/10.1186/
1471-2458-10-533

30. Kulwicki, A. & Hill Rice, V. Arab
American adolescent perceptions and
experiences with smoking. *Public Health
Nursing.* 2003;20(3):177–83. https://doi
.org/10.1046/j.0737-1209.2003.20304.x

31. Alsuwaidi, A. R., Hammad, H. A. A. K.,
Elbarazi, I., & Sheek-Hussein, M. Vaccine
hesitancy within the Muslim community:
Islamic faith and public health
perspectives. *Human Vaccines and
Immunotherapeutics.* 2023;19(1):1–7.
https://doi.org/10.1080/21645515.2023
.2190716

32. Ammar, N., Couture-Carron, A., Alvi, S.,
& Antonio, J. S. Experiences of Muslim
and Non-Muslim battered immigrant
women with the police in the United
States: a closer understanding of
commonalities and differences. *Violence
Against Women.* 2013;19(12):1449–71.
https://doi.org/10.1177/
1077801213517565

33. Sapry, H. R. & Takiudin, N. S.
Challenges faced by non-Muslim
transporter in adopting *halal* logistics
certificate. *Journal of Critical Reviews.*
2023;7(8):141–46.

34. Wibowo, M. W., Permana, D., Hanafiah,
A., Ahmad, F. S., & Ting, H. *Halal*
food credence: do the Malaysian non-
Muslim consumers hesitate? *Journal of
Islamic Marketing.* 2021;12(8):1405–24.
https://doi.org/10.1108/JIMA-01-2020-0013

35. Sukhabot, S. & Jumani, Z. A. Islamic
brands attitudes and its consumption
behaviour among non-Muslim residents
of Thailand. *Journal of Islamic Marketing.*
2023;14(1):196–214. https://doi.org/10
.1108/JIMA-05-2021-0155

36. Ustadi, M. N., Osman, S., & Rasi, R. Z.
Perception of non-Muslim manufacturers
towards *halal* food supply chain in
Malaysia. *International Journal of*

Innovation, Creativity, and Change. 2020;10(11):430–40.

37. Iranmanesh, M., Senali, M. G., Ghobakhloo, M., Nikbin, D., & Ghazanfar, A. A. Customer behaviour towards *halal* food: a systematic review and agenda for future research. *Journal of Islamic Marketing.* 2022;13(9):1901–17. https://doi.org/10.1108/JIMA-01-2021-0031

Chapter 25

Challenges and Solutions in Public Health: An Islamic Perspective

Joshua Bernstein

Introduction

The goal of the worldwide public health community is to protect and improve the health and well-being of populations on global, regional, and community scales. This includes a broad range of efforts developed to prevent disease, promote health, and increase equitable access to health care and health-related resources for all people regardless of geographic location or socioeconomic status [1]. These goals often include measurable objectives such as disease monitoring and response, developing and maintaining health care infrastructure, conducting and sharing new research, and developing and implementing policies on disease prevention, treatment, health maintenance, emergency response, and global collaboration.

In global Muslim communities, the concept of public health is closely aligned with the teachings and principles of Islam. Islamic teachings emphasize the importance of taking care of one's health and the well-being of the community, acknowledging the interconnectedness of physical, mental, and spiritual health, and, in all endeavors, moving closer to God (Allah). The Holy Qur'an contains principles and guidance that can be interpreted as emphasizing public health [2]. While the Holy Qur'an doesn't explicitly discuss modern concepts of public health, many of its teachings are relevant to promoting well-being, hygiene, and communal responsibility [2]. This could be understood as per the history of the development of medicine and public health terminology after the early eighth through thirteenth centuries, known as the Islamic Golden Age. Hence, preventing disease occurrence has always been considered better than treating it, as reflected by the Islamic public health messages.

In the global Muslim communities, the concept of public health is closely aligned with the teachings and principles of Islam. The Muslim community often integrates spiritual and religious aspects into health practices. Western public health, on the other hand, may be more secular in its approach, focusing primarily on scientific and evidence-based strategies, and it may actively avoid or remove spirituality as a health care consideration [3]. For example, the Islamic faith can influence practices such as dietary habits, personal hygiene, and fasting as instructed in the Holy Qur'an: "*O ye who believe! Fasting is prescribed to you as it was prescribed to those before you, that ye may (learn) self-restraint*" (Q Al-Baqarah 2:183), whereas a Western model may ignore or remove these influences from a treatment or prevention plan. Social, cultural, and sexual influences also interact with public health policy and practice in Muslim communities [4].

The Islamic and Western public health models share many goals and objectives. However, specific differences must be acknowledged and understood. To date, there is no global approach that operates effectively within these cultures. Public health practitioners require a working understanding of the unique elements within Muslim communities that affect the development, promotion, application, and maintenance of public health issues [5].

Public Health in the Twenty-First Century

Modern public health is shaped by a variety of factors, including advancements in technology, changes in global demographics, evolving health threats, and a growing recognition of the importance of addressing social determinants of health. Developed and developing nations are moving towards a systems-based approach to health and well-being. Public health in the twenty-first century recognizes that preventive measures and health outcomes are influenced by social, economic, and environmental factors [6]. However, these factors may or may not incorporate sociocultural and religious norms, beliefs, practices, and expectations. Additionally, with the rapid spread of information online, including the prevalence of misinformation, effective health communication is critical. Public health agencies use various channels to provide accurate information, raise awareness, and educate the public about health risks and preventive measures. Yet in some societies and cultures individuals and communities get much of their health information from cultural and religious organizations. The Muslim community values information and directions found in the Holy Qur'an, the Hadith, and local or regional spiritual leaders [7]. While there is value in these sources, some information may contradict contemporary public health knowledge and practice. As a result, public health policies and norms may be influenced by a blend of religious beliefs, cultural traditions, and scientific knowledge.

Public health behaviors in Muslim societies have been historically affected by religious beliefs, cultural practices, and local contexts. Islam places great importance on the well-being of individuals and communities, and, as a result, many public health norms in Muslim regions align with Islamic teachings [8]. With this regard, instructions on seeking healthy practices, cures, and medications were advocated by the Prophet Muhammad (PBUH), as he said, "Seek remedies, O people. For God has not placed any disease without making for it a cure, except one illness: old age" [9]. However, practices and interpretations can vary across different Muslim-majority countries and communities. Public health and health promotion agencies must demonstrate cultural understanding and proficiency when interacting with Muslim individuals and communities as well as at the regional policy level [2]. Health issues associated with epidemic control and vaccination, safety and sanitation, dietary practices, and individual treatment options must be viewed contextually if the goal is understanding, adoption, and practice. In the near future, public health will be inextricably linked to emerging technologies, and developing regions are at risk of not receiving the full benefits of these contemporary practices. A blended approach that retains historic culture and tradition and includes modern methodologies is needed.

Health Challenges in Muslim Societies

Public health issues vary based on geographic location, cultural and socioeconomic factors, and the specific circumstances of different communities. For Muslims, like any other religious or cultural group, important public health issues can include a range of concerns that share commonalities with the global population in addition to specifics within their unique society. In conventional Muslim regions, there are distinct environmental challenges that can complicate public health initiatives such as health care access, clean drinking water, sanitation, health literacy, and factors associated with migrants and refugees [8]. These health and health-related issues can be differentiated based on socioeconomic status, cultural practices within Muslim individuals and communities, and the current sociopolitical status of a region. Addressing these public health concerns requires collaboration between health care providers, policymakers, religious leaders, and community organizations to develop culturally appropriate and effective interventions [2]. Muslim political leaders, spiritual advisors, and community members must be involved in the public health planning, implementation, and evaluation cycle.

Predicting specific public health challenges over the next 10 years in Muslim societies involves a significant degree of uncertainty, particularly when faced with addressing the United Nations Sustainable Development Goals. However, based on ongoing trends and emerging global issues, several potential challenges and issues could arise. Similar to European and Western societies, Muslims should encounter increased exposure to emerging infectious diseases due to gradual urbanization, climate change, and cultural changes (e.g., adopting some elements of Western culture) [6]. Noncommunicable diseases present a significant public health challenge given some contemporary public health practices may conflict with cultural and religious practice. Public health practitioners should look for common ground between these two institutions versus how they might compete. Additionally, with an aging population, the prevalence of mental health issues, barriers to health care access and equity, and debilitating illnesses will increase [10]. Furthermore, as the global public health community increasingly relies on modern medical integration, education, health literacy, and data-driven technologies, the traditional/regional Muslim communities – largely rural and agrarian – may be slow to benefit from this progress [10]. Introducing these elements into a traditional Muslim society should be done carefully, systematically, and in consultation with community and spiritual leaders.

Public Health Opportunities

Undertaking positive change and continuous development are highly promoted in Islam, as the Holy Qur'an in Q Ar-Ra'd 13:11 states: *"Allah does not change the condition of a people until they change what is within themselves. And if Allah wills hardship for a people there is no turning it back, and there is no protector for them but Allah."* This could serve as the basis of the numerous successful public health initiatives that have been implemented in Muslim societies to address a range of health challenges. These initiatives often leverage a combination of local knowledge, cultural sensitivity, and evidence-based approaches. Pakistan made significant progress in polio eradication through innovative strategies [11]. Their program included community engagement, the use of local religious leaders to promote vaccination, and the adaption of vaccination campaigns that accommodated religious practices and cultural norms. Public health professionals built this successful program using a collaborative model that empowered cultural and religious stakeholders. In Afghanistan, lay community health workers were trained to provide basic health care services to underserved areas, particularly in rural and conflict-affected regions, that allowed unique access to communities, families, and individuals who were either unable or unwilling to seek contemporary health care services [12]. Saudi Arabia has implemented large-scale water and sanitation projects to improve access to clean water and sanitation facilities in both urban and rural areas [13]. These efforts have reduced waterborne diseases and improved overall health. This policy-driven initiative began with health education messages congruent with regional culture and religious practice. Community acceptance was sought prior to and during the planning and implementation phases of this public health project.

Unsuccessful public health initiatives can result from various factors, including inadequate planning, lack of community engagement, cultural insensitivity, or challenges in implementation rooted in a lack of understanding, acceptance, and community empowerment [14]. The right message, policy, or practice can be predicted to struggle or fail when top-down or outside initiatives attempt to dictate what should be done and how. In Pakistan, a measles vaccination campaign faced significant challenges due to vaccine hesitancy [15]. The initial efforts produced misinformation and concerns about the vaccine's safety. Similarly, in some Muslim-majority areas in northern Nigeria, health professionals experienced considerable resistance to polio vaccination campaigns due to misconceptions, rumors, and distrust of Western medicine [16]. This led to a resurgence of polio cases in the region and underscored the importance of community engagement and cultural sensitivity that was missing in the original program plan. In Afghanistan, initiatives developed to educate girls and women about reproductive health faced significant challenges due to cultural norms that limited girls' education and discouraged discussions about sexuality [17]. Without guidance and support from local cultural and religious leaders, the program was unsuccessful.

Similar to program planning and implementation at the community level, top-down legislative and policy solutions should be sensitive to cultural, religious, and social contexts [18]. These ideas should aim to address the unique health challenges faced by Muslim communities while promoting equitable and inclusive health care. Legislative efforts should consider culturally competent health services that integrate modern, evidence-based practices. This can be done using a variety of approaches that may include:

Health Care Services: Develop guidelines and standards for health care providers to ensure culturally competent care for Muslim patients. This includes training health care professionals in religious practices, dietary restrictions, and modesty considerations.

Health Advocates: Collaborate with religious leaders to promote health awareness and education in alignment with Islamic teachings. Religious leaders can help dispel myths, encourage preventive measures, and support health campaigns.

Community and Lay Health Workers: Train community health workers within Muslim communities to serve as intermediaries between health care systems and community members. These lay community workers can provide culturally sensitive health education and support.

Food and Nutrition Education: Implement policies that ensure the availability of *halal* food in health care facilities and schools. Additionally, promote nutrition education that aligns with Islamic dietary guidelines and combines contemporary nutrition guidelines with culturally congruent religious tradition.

Immunization Outreach: Collaborate with religious leaders to endorse and promote vaccination campaigns, using religious teachings to emphasize the importance of protecting health through immunization.

Health Education: Form cooperative agreements with Islamic educational institutions to incorporate health education into curricula, covering topics such as hygiene, nutrition, and disease prevention.

Research Reporting: Support research initiatives that focus on public health challenges specific to Muslim communities and that are conducted by Muslims in collaboration with non-Muslim institutions who can promote culturally sensitive data collection, analysis, and reporting.

Policy initiatives should be adapted to the unique needs and contexts of each Muslim-majority region, country, or community. They should also involve collaboration with community members, religious leaders, health care professionals, and policymakers to promote effective implementation and maintenance.

Conclusion

The global Muslim community can and should coexist with modern public health practice while maintaining its traditional identity, spiritual foundation, and culture. A mixed approach to current and near-future public health issues should incorporate contemporary research and practice in harmony with an understanding of the Islamic culture and belief system. Top-down legislative efforts and grassroots, community-level initiatives should begin collaboratively. Public health professionals, cultural and spiritual leaders, and members of a target community should work together to assess public health needs, plan new initiatives or evaluate current programs, and implement these strategies.

References

1. World Health Organization. What we do. [online]. 2022 [Accessed May 2, 2023]. Available from: www.who.int/about/what-we-do

2. El-Hamdoon, O. E. Islam and public health. *Journal of the British Islamic Medical Association*. 2021;8(3):1–4.

3. Chamsi-Pasha, H. & Ali Albar, M. Western and Islamic bioethics: how close is the gap? *Avicenna Journal of Medicine*. 2013;3(1):8–14. https://doi.org/10.4103/2231-0770.112788

4. Padela, A. I. & Curlin, F. A. Religion and disparities: considering the influences of Islam on the health of American Muslims. *Journal of Religion and Health*. 2013;52:1333–45. https://doi.org/10.1007/s10943-012-9620-y

5. World Health Organization. Health promotion. [online]. 2021 [Accessed May 2, 2023]. Available from: www.who.int/health-topics/health-promotion#tab=tab_1

6. Chatelan, A. & Khalatbari-Soltani, S. Evaluating and rethinking public health for the 21st century: toward vulnerable population interventions. *Frontiers in Public Health*. 2022;10:1033270. https://doi.org/10.3389/fpubh.2022.1033270

7. Ismail, W. M., Al-Mushaiqri, M. R. S., & Haiyan, L. Inclusion of Islamic peace concepts in school curricula. *Journal of Dharma*. 2021;46:501–16.

8. Koenig, H. G. & Al Shohaib, S. *Health and Well-Being in Islamic Societies: Background, Research, and Applications*. New York: Springer. 2014.

9. Sunan Ibn Majah. *Sunan Ibn Majah 3436*. In-book reference: Book 31, Hadith 1. Available from: https://sunnah.com/ibnmajah:3436

10. Yunus, R. M. Public health: an Islamic perspective. *International Journal of Islamic Thoughts*. 2017;6(2):69–82.

11. Hussain, S. F., Boyle, P., Patel, P., & Sullivan, R. Eradicating polio in Pakistan: an analysis of the challenges and solutions to this security and health issue.

Globalization and Health. 2016;12 (63). https://doi.org/10.1186/s12992-016-0195-3

12. Najafizada, S. A. M., Labonte, R., & Bourgeault, I. L. Community health workers of Afghanistan: a qualitative study of a national program. *Conflict and Health.* 2014;8(26). https://doi.org/10.1186/1752-1505-8-26

13. Gazzeh, K. & Abubakar, I. R. Regional disparity in access to basic public services in Saudi Arabia: a sustainability challenge. *Utilities Policy.* 2018;52:70–80. https://doi.org/10.1016/j.jup.2018.04.008

14. Abd Rahman, A. & Mahmud, A. A Review of the Islamic approach in public health practices. *International Journal of Public Health and Clinical Science.* 2014;1(2):2289–7577.

15. Khowaja, A. R., Khan, S. A., Nizam, N., Omer, S. B., & Zaidi, A. Parental perceptions surrounding polio and self-reported non-participation in polio supplementary immunization activities in Karachi, Pakistan: a mixed methods study. *World Health Organization.* 2012;90:822–30. https://doi.org/10.2471/blt.12.106260

16. Abdulraheem, I. S., Onajole, A. T, & Oladipo, A. Reasons for incomplete vaccination and factors for missed opportunities among rural Nigerian children. *Journal of Public Health Epidemiology.* 2011;3:194–203.

17. UNICEF. Education: providing quality education for all. [online]. n.d. [Accessed May 2, 2023]. Available from: www.unicef.org/afghanistan/education

18. Esquierdo-Leal, J. L. & Houmanfar, R. A. Creating inclusive and equitable cultural practices by linking leadership to systemic change. *Behavior Analysis in Practice.* 2021;14(2):499–512. https://doi.org/10.1007/s40617-020-00519-7

Index

Printed in the United States
by Baker & Taylor Publisher Services